Caregiver Family Therapy

Caregiver Family Therapy

Empowering Families to Meet the Challenges of Aging

Sara Honn Qualls and Ashley A. Williams

American Psychological Association • Washington, DC

Published by
American Psychological Association
750 First Street, NE
Washington, DC 20002
www.apa.org

To order
APA Order Department
P.O. Box 92984
Washington, DC 20090-2984
Tel: (800) 374-2721; Direct: (202) 336-5510
Fax: (202) 336-5502; TDD/TTY: (202) 336-6123
Online: www.apa.org/pubs/books
E-mail: order@apa.org

In the U.K., Europe, Africa, and the Middle East, copies may be ordered from
American Psychological Association
3 Henrietta Street
Covent Garden, London
WC2E 8LU England

Typeset in Meridien by Circle Graphics, Inc., Columbia, MD

Printer: Maple Press, York, PA
Cover Designer: Mercury Publishing Services, Rockville, MD

The opinions and statements published are the responsibility of the authors, and such opinions and statements do not necessarily represent the policies of the American Psychological Association.

Library of Congress Cataloging-in-Publication Data

Qualls, Sarah Honn.
 Caregiver family therapy : empowering families to meet the challenges of aging / Sara Honn
 Qualls and Ashley A. Williams.
   p. cm.
 Includes bibliographical references and index.
 ISBN 978-1-4338-1214-9 — ISBN 1-4338-1214-2 1. Caregivers. 2. Care of the sick—Psychological
aspects. 3. Older people—Care. 4. Family therapy. I. Williams, Ashley A. II. Title.

 RA645.3.Q83 2013
 362.1—dc23
                                        2012013750

British Library Cataloguing-in-Publication Data
A CIP record is available from the British Library.

Printed in the United States of America
First Edition

DOI: 10.1037/13943-000

*Dedicated to our future caregivers
Morgan, Lea, and Marcus Qualls
and
Zachary and Zeke Williams*

Contents

Preface

Family members often struggle to figure out how to care well for each other, especially when an older member becomes ill or disabled. For over a decade, we and other clinicians in the Aging Families and Caregiver Program at the University of Colorado (CU) Aging Center have been trying to help older adults and their families navigate through very challenging moments in this phase of the family life cycle. During this time, our framework for treating caregiving families has evolved through many versions, thanks to the invaluable contributions of many clinicians-in-training, staff, and faculty.

The first time we were challenged to articulate our treatment approach was in 2006. At that time, we had a general treatment approach but had not outlined it as a formal model. To prepare for being featured in an American Psychological Association (APA) training video for working with families dealing with Alzheimer's disease, we had to articulate our model. The first time we met to do so, we stared at each other with that blank look that is common among clinicians who work more intuitively than prescriptively. However, as the group took up the challenge, we were pleasantly surprised to find that we really were relatively systematic in our approach to assessment and intervention with caregiving families.

Several years after that first effort to articulate the model (APA, 2006), a cohort of doctoral trainees worked on a modular version (Anderson et al., 2008). Their version of the model was more complex and better suited to meet the needs of the wide range of caregivers and aging families who ask for help in community-based programs. The modules that our trainees outlined formed the foundation of our current model, although the current model is organized not as a linear progression but as a repeating circular sequence of issues that caregivers address and readdress over time. Over the past 2 years, the clinical team has revised the trainees' framework and articulated the intervention strategies more consistently. When it was time to write a full description of caregiver family therapy (CFT) that could serve as a therapy guidebook or manual, the two of us (Qualls and Williams) took on that project. This book is our first effort to extend the CFT model beyond the principles that could be articulated in a chapter (Qualls, 2008; Qualls & Noecker, 2009), with clinical examples and suggested strategies.

The evolution of the model has been a shared labor of love over a 12-year period, engaging supervisors, therapists, and trainees at the CU Aging Center. This unique center is a university-operated training clinic located in a community senior services complex. Services are provided either free or on a sliding scale basis and are thus available to all (however, Medicare reimbursement is not available for work provided by trainees). The CU Aging Center has maintained a contract with the Pikes Peak Area Agency on Aging (AAA) to provide caregiver counseling services funded by the Older Americans Act. The AAA's colleagueship, support, and collaboration over the years have contributed significantly to our ideas and practices. Yet, the heavy lifting has been done by trainees, staff, and supervisors. They are the ones who have developed innovative strategies, critiqued our ideas, tested our suggestions in the therapy room, and made their work available for us to consider together. We are eternally grateful for having such outstanding colleagues and students who are allowing us to be the authorship voice of this model at the moment. Some of them will elaborate the model and extend our ideas in research and clinical scholarship far beyond this initial statement, and we anticipate their work with joy and appreciation.

Caregiver
Family
Therapy

Introduction

D uring the 20th century, the average life expectancy in the
United States increased by 30 years, from 47 to approximately 79 (World Health Organization, 2011). Every component of our society has been affected by that change, and
none shows the impact more dramatically than families.
Increasingly, family members must provide care for older
adults with physical or cognitive impairments. Whether the
impairments are a result of stroke, dementia, or chronic illness, the burdens of caregiving can put significant strain on
caregivers and their relationships with other family members and loved ones, including the care recipient.

The needs of caregiving families are varied and complex,
as is reflected in the myriad reasons why family members
seek help from therapists, aging centers, social services,
medical providers, senior housing providers, and other providers. These reasons include, for example, a fear of what
lies ahead, frustration that the care recipient does not cooperate with needed changes, conflict among family members about key decisions, and burnout or depression in the

DOI: 10.1037/13943-010
Caregiver Family Therapy: Empowering Families to Meet the Challenges of Aging,
by S. H. Qualls and A. A. Williams

primary caregiver. Family members may want help talking with an older member to explore feelings about care options, to address difficult care concerns (e.g., driving), or to validate the person's right to quit the never-ending list of possible treatments that can at best delay death for a short period. Furthermore, family members can seek help at any stage of caregiving, from the early precaregiving stage, when family-care patterns are similar to previous life phases, to postdeath of the older adult, when caregiving relationship structures are relinquished and family relationships realigned.

Caregiver family therapy (CFT) is a treatment model that offers a framework for addressing these and other complex needs of families caring for older adults. Specifically, CFT guides families through the developmental transitions of later life. It helps members figure out exactly what changes have occurred in the older adult care recipient, adapt family roles to meet the needs of that older adult, and ensure that the caregiver and other family members have structured caregiving roles in a way that can be sustained without undue cost to the well-being of any family member. Therapists work with one or more members of the family to create family-level shifts in roles that position families to meet the needs of an older adult whose illness or disability has positioned him or her as a recipient of care.

Usually there are many involved family members spread across thousands of miles. Sometimes, the older adult who is the target of concern does not participate in the therapy because he or she lacks either the capacity or the willingness to do so. Other times, the older person is continuously engaged in the treatment. Across these variations, the commonality is that the therapist must join one or more members of the frightened family, respect their very long history, and assist them in sorting out what to do and how to do it.

Three Core Processes, Three Main Points for Intervention

CFT focuses on the three most distressing processes, or stages, of family caregiving: addressing the care recipient's problem, establishing the caregiving role structures, and addressing the caregiver's self-care. Therapists can determine which process may be most distressing to a particular family member by listening to the language describing the presenting problem. Examples of common problem reports that focus on the care recipient include statements such as the following:

- "He just won't do anything to help himself."
- "She is so mean to the staff that I'm afraid the facility is going to kick her out."

- "My mother's true self is emerging now that she is demented—she swears like a sailor and tries to get in bed with every man on the unit."
- "My dad refuses to see a doctor, so how am I supposed to get him the help he needs?"
- "Would you treat my mother for depression? She just won't do any of the things she has always enjoyed."

Caregivers who use language focusing on the care structures may describe problems in the relationship between caregiver and care recipient, among family members, between family and other care systems, or between care recipient and other care systems. Examples of presenting problems that focus on role structures include the following:

- "My dad will do anything my brother asks but won't do a damn thing for me, and I'm the one who is supposed to be taking care of him."
- "My mother simply won't take charge of my father even though she knows he is incapable of making his own decisions."
- "My wife has a serious alcohol problem but insists on caring for her mother."
- "The doctor won't approve hospice, but my father is refusing to eat so is killing himself."
- "My sister is a physician at Harvard, so Daddy listens to her when she says I am making too much of the problem, but she doesn't see his day-to-day problems."
- "My teenagers are driving me crazy, just at the time that my parents need so much attention."
- "We need to take away her car keys, but we have no idea how to do that."
- "The assisted living facility insists that mother needs to be in their dementia unit, but I think that moving her there will kill her."

Caregivers who use language focusing on themselves may say they are depressed or anxious as a result of the ongoing burden of caregiving, or they may anticipate changes in their capacity to maintain existing roles because of new family responsibilities (e.g., remarriage, travel, relocation). Presenting statements focusing on caregiver self-care include the following:

- "I just can't do this anymore; I am so worn out that I can't sleep or eat."
- "My kids never see me anymore, and that's not fair to them."
- "My doctor said I needed to see you because my blood pressure just keeps rising."
- "I'm being transferred across country—who will oversee Mom's care now?"

- "This is a peak time in my career responsibilities. Am I just selfish to want to succeed even if it means I can't visit Mom every day?"
- "I haven't exercised in months—there just isn't time."
- "I can't leave him alone so how could I possibly go out with my friends?"
- "Fun—what is that?"
- "My boss talked to me about all of my trips to care for my parents with sympathy but made it clear that I can't continue this pattern of being gone for a week every few months."

Regardless of which process the presenting family member finds most distressing when therapy begins, each core process is ultimately addressed in CFT, because the processes repeat in a cyclical fashion throughout the caregiving journey. Each process is a stage of adaptation that occurs at multiple points in the caregiving journey. The content of each stage varies, but all stages involve the therapist asking questions and engaging the caregivers in change. In this sense, the stages are remarkably similar in our experience. No single right answer or approach exists to providing care for frail older adults, even among those in the same stage of caregiving. However, we assert that asking the same questions will guide the family toward choices that support the well-being of all involved.

Overview of CFT

In Figure 1, the core set of adaptation processes used in CFT is depicted as three points of a triangle: naming the problem, role structuring, and caregiver self-care. Transition processes along the sides of the triangle flow automatically from the core processes. These transition processes include "structuring care" through problem solving, checking the impact of role structures (or "role reverberations") on the primary caregiver's overall well-being as well as on other family members, and "widening the lens" to consider any broader implications of the situation. We position the adaptation processes around a circle to illustrate the ongoing, cyclical nature of adaptation that occurs and reoccurs at each phase of the caregiving journey. However, families do not feel like they have taken a massive turn around the tip of a triangle when they resolve challenges at one point of the triangle; their experience is far more continuous and thus better represented by a circle.

We envision a CFT episode as engaging the clients in this full cycle, with the potential for repeating it in future episodes of CFT when the care situation and the caregivers' needs warrant. In other words, caregiving families seek help for the particular needs of the moment. The

FIGURE 1

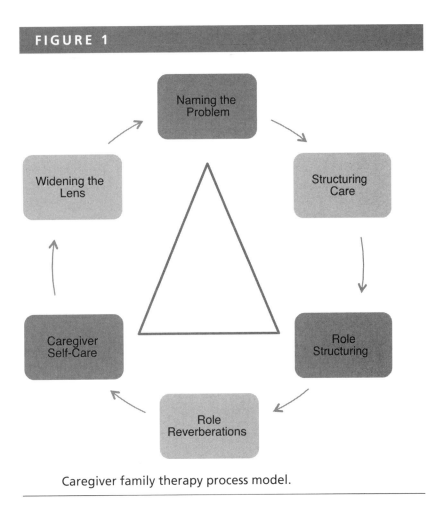

Caregiver family therapy process model.

full cycle of work for the current situation involves accurately naming this problem, configuring roles for this situation, and ensuring that the caregiver is engaging in adequate self-care for this moment in time. The cycle may take only one or two sessions if the family is already well adapted to a well-known situation and simply needs reassurance or referral to specific providers. Other families will use several sessions spread over many weeks or months to complete a full trip around the circle as it relates to their current care situation. Furthermore, as the care recipients' functioning changes over time, some families will return to work on the needs of future moments. Others will be able to use the knowledge, skills, and resources gained in one cycle of work to adapt to future needs on their own.

The processes we define as core to CFT are obviously not unique to this model. However, our systems approach leads us to conduct what we refer to as "impact checks" after each step, to check for collateral damage or opportunities that this work might have created. We recognize that caregivers live in complex family and community systems that are inevitably going to be affected by any change in the role of any individual. We end a sequence of work by widening the lens to look at possible effects of our intervention on the larger family system, to ensure that caregivers' roles are not deleteriously affecting the development of other members of the system.

Future Directions

We recognize several very important steps that lie ahead in the development of the CFT model. First and foremost, empirical tests of the value of the model are needed. Although clinical experience supports the model, efficacy studies have not yet been conducted. Flexible models like this one are challenging to test because they offer the intervention to a very wide variety of consumers across diverse settings. Assessment of the impact of the intervention will be challenging but must be done to test its value. Tools to direct therapy and to assess each step of the process model are needed, along with determination of whether different strategies are needed for assessing them at different stages of caregiving.

Of equal importance with scientific tests of the effectiveness of CFT are questions about the applicability of the model across different cultural groups. We recognize that CFT was developed in a particular sociocultural context and thus will have boundaries on its applicability. We do not yet understand those boundaries because we have attempted to create a principled approach that can adapt to a wide range of cultural groups. However, we anticipate that others will see the limitations that are not yet visible to us and will help either adapt the model or define its limitations.

This Volume

This volume was written to guide clinicians and counselors in implementing CFT. Grounded in research on caregiving families' challenges, existing family therapy models, and, where possible, evidence-based protocols, the book provides detailed strategies for assessment and intervention. The majority of the strategies have been developed in our clinic, the University of Colorado (CU) Aging Center, and tested with numerous caregivers served by many different clinicians. That variation in providers and clients has been a valuable proving ground to teach us what works for almost everyone and which approaches are creative adaptations that rely on a particular clinician's personality or style.

Chapter 1 discusses the empirical and theoretical foundations of CFT. Chapters 2 through 7 discuss each stage of CFT sequentially, including the three core stages and the three transition stages. Brief clinical examples appear as exhibits in each stage chapter to illustrate the nearly infinite variations in caregiving family styles, challenges, and solutions. Chapter 8 presents two in-depth case studies illustrating how the steps of CFT unfold. The first case follows Linda and her family as they deal with her mother's declining cognitive abilities, and the second follows Lupé and her husband, Julio, as they navigate the spouse caregiving journey for chronic physical health conditions. Chapter 9 addresses practical issues in delivering CFT in various settings, including ethical and business issues as well as practical issues in implementing therapy. Finally, two appendices provide additional resources for clinicians. Appendix A presents the Caregiver Reaction Scale, an instrument used in the CU Aging Center to assess how family members are coping with the caregiving role, including both positive and negative effects. Appendix B is a one-page summary of the CFT process that clinicians can photocopy for quick reference.

Although this book is primarily written for therapists, we also recognize the value of CFT for other service providers. Many providers in senior housing, social services, health care, or legal services are not positioned to contract with families for a therapeutic intervention, yet are well positioned to support family adaptation to care transitions. Many providers are in the position to use a simple intervention to calm an agitated family who is absorbing inordinate amounts of staff time in senior housing or help a family move forward with difficult decisions, like taking away car keys. We have tried to make our description of this model accessible to a range of professionals who want to help family caregivers succeed in adapting to the extraordinary family shifts required along this challenging path. Ultimately, we hope this volume will help numerous providers guide families in their caregiving journey.

Foundations of Caregiver Family Therapy

1

Caregiving for aging members is an increasingly prevalent and potent experience for families that affects their very structure and function. After suggesting parameters for defining a caregiving family, this chapter overviews the journey of caregiving for a person with chronic disease. We then describe the state of the literature on existing caregiving interventions and argue for the importance of addressing family structures and functioning, offering a distinct family therapy approach we call *caregiver family therapy* (CFT). Finally, we describe the unique features and theoretical foundations of CFT.

Elder Care Hits the Family System

Past generations of caregivers have approached care for elder family members by following examples set by their family members and friends. New family structures and cultural

DOI: 10.1037/13943-001
Caregiver Family Therapy: Empowering Families to Meet the Challenges of Aging,
by S. H. Qualls and A. A. Williams

contexts have emerged during recent decades, and these have dramatically shifted approaches to caregiving.

NEW FAMILY STRUCTURES

Families of the 21st century experience aging in entirely different contexts from previous generations within their lineage. Families are dealing with greater longevity and totally different social–political–economic contexts. Consider the following experiences that an additional 3 decades of the life span creates for families (Blieszner, 2009):

- Most adults can now expect to be parents three times as long as they were children.
- Siblings' relationships span approximately 80 years.
- Most adults will have parents over age 60 longer than they will have children in their home.
- Midlife adults will have more aging parents than they have children.
- Women are almost certain to spend time living alone in adulthood.

The structure of intergenerational families has shifted from a branching tree to a beanpole (Hagestad, 1986; see Figure 1.1). Increasingly, three generations are alive simultaneously, with four- and five-generation families occurring for brief periods (Blieszner, 2009). Although the number of vertical relationships (across generations) has grown in the past century, the fertility rates have declined, yielding

FIGURE 1.1

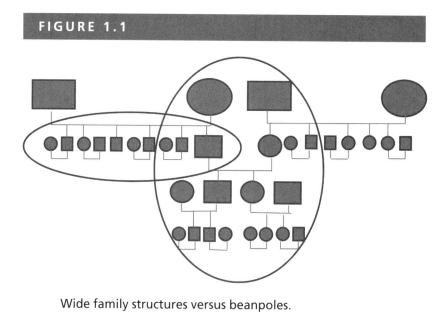

Wide family structures versus beanpoles.

fewer members of each generation—hence the beanpole image of tall, skinny family trees with layers of intergenerational relationships and few intragenerational relationships.

Fewer siblings, cousins, aunts, and uncles means fewer people to share the workload of care for the bookend members of the family. Children and elderly people are the frailest members of any society, yet they also engage in mutual caregiving characteristics of families. Grandparents rear grandchildren when parents cannot manage, at least in part because there often are no aunts or uncles to incorporate the children into their homes. Those grandparents may also be caring for their parents because elder care responsibilities fall on that same bean-pole lineage as the need arises. Even young children care for frail parents, grandparents, and great-grandparents, supplementing others' caregiving roles or taking on the full responsibility early in life (Shifren, 2008). Whereas siblings had the option of sharing child care or parent care in previous eras, today the responsibilities are usually off-loaded either up or down the family beanpole. As a result, modern families must not only provide care for older adults but also do so without having seen previous generations do so. Lacking examples from their own youth, most families caring for older adults must "make it up as they go."

NEW CULTURAL CONTEXTS

Across ethnic groups and family structures, considerable variability is evident in the roles assigned to family and paid providers (Knight & Sayegh, 2010; National Alliance for Caregiving, 2011). Many families who immigrated in the past 100 years have very different experiences of acculturation across the generations that influence expectations about the aging experience and caregiving. First-generation immigrants are likely to acculturate far less fully than their children and grandchildren. Those from cultures that emphasize familism over individualism may be particularly prone to generationally based values conflicts as later generations adopt more individualistic values and lifestyles while aging family members expect familistic values and structures for caregiving (Losada et al., 2010).

The social environment in which families care for their elders also has shifted dramatically over the past century. The current generation of elderly adults is the wealthiest ever to live, with enormous financial capital to invest in maintaining their independence as long as possible. Social Security and Medicare added safety nets that allow families to expect elderly members to live separately using their own financial resources. However, public social service systems have not kept pace with private wealth development, so the safety net is lower to the ground than most families expect. Furthermore, families whose income or assets are just above the threshold for qualifying for safety net services, such as Medicaid, find their options remarkably limited. Chronic, long-term care is where the service gaps are experienced most dramatically (Fingerman, Miller, & Seidel, 2009).

The health care industry accounts for 16.2% of the economy (Global Health Observatory, 2009), in sharp contrast to the family doctor who made house calls in 1900 as a cottage industry. Most of us are daunted by the complexity of the systems of care, insurance, and range of providers we see in the course of a year. Older adults are the heaviest users of the health care system, but the system is not easy for them (or anyone else) to navigate. Families of older adults continue to be their primary health care support team members, providing the vast majority of the supportive care that they need, so they are inevitably involved in their health care. Yet families are in the awkward position of being the official responsible party who is expected to arrive to handle emergencies even though they lack access to medical records or the privilege of collaborating with the rest of the team.

Health conditions are also more complex today. Older people likely had the same range of diseases and disorders a century ago, but without a way to measure or see them, fewer labels were applied, fewer assessments were ordered, and fewer treatments prescribed. Families did not have to distinguish between the effects of intravenous hydration versus feeding tubes, the funding options for medical rehabilitation versus strengthening exercises, or services options such as hospice and palliative care, as just three examples among myriad real situations likely to face a family on a given day. Elder care often places families right in the middle of the extraordinarily complex, highly technical health care world with no time to get the background training needed to participate effectively.

The power structures in health care are shifting. A century ago, physicians had more decision-making rights than patients or families. Today, patients' rights are increasingly being defined and legally protected. Families are the group whose rights have still not been well defined. Patients can choose treatments that place demands on families without consulting their families. Insurance companies also have power over our health never envisioned a century ago, constraining or supplying services that have a direct impact on families.

Housing options for older adults have exploded in the past 3 decades, especially as older adults implemented their desire to live separately from family members. After living independently for 80 years, many older men and women who need a simpler, more supportive environment are not interested in moving in with children. Nor are many of them willing to go to nursing homes. Congregate living facilities evolved into campuses with multiple levels of care. Assisted living became the preferred choice for frail persons. Nursing homes became highly medicalized settings with little that resembles a home still visible.

Home-based services have emerged to support older adults who need limited assistance in order to live in their own homes. Because these services are organized idiosyncratically in each community, they are not simple to access. Services include transportation, meals, case management, personal care, and home care, among others. The funding streams supporting these programs grew, shrank, changed form, and in most cases became more difficult to access. At the same time, new programs such as the Program for All-Inclusive Care for the Elderly developed to address the exploding costs of nursing-home care borne by the states while supporting aging-in-place by very frail older adults (Mukamel et al., 2006).

In short, the cultural contexts of aging have evolved so rapidly that our great-grandparents would be as shocked by the current social and health services structures as they would be by rocket ships. Family caregivers may feel like they have to learn rocket science in order to navigate these systems effectively.

No Simple Solution

Although many caregiving tasks are practical and manageable, some of the problems faced by aging families have no simple solution even for those of us who work inside these systems. Technology has advanced far faster than has the evolution of our emotion–thought centers involved in life-and-death decisions. Ethics boards exist in hospitals to help clarify the complexities in health care so that families as well as patients and health providers can at least see the values choices facing them. Some problems have no simple answers and thus require us to make very difficult decisions without any authority figure pointing the way (see the example in Exhibit 1.1).

Another reason that solutions are not simple for families is that they cannot look to previous generations for guidance on how to navigate the systems or how to prioritize care options. The changing contexts of aging mean that the ways in which previous generations struggled with values clashes over caregiving are also hard to apply to current situations. Aging is a whole new world for this generation of family caregivers.

The impact of our family members' aging on our life structure, family, and core identity is huge. As one of us (SHQ) has often commented, "My perspective on myself and my family changed forever when I first diapered my mother." Something profound happens when members of your own generation or those ahead of you fully depend on you for care. Something profound also happens when you become the care

EXHIBIT 1.1

Jim

Jim hates his life in assisted living and desperately wants his own apartment again. He is confident that he can drive safely, despite the effects of the stroke. Neuropsychological evaluations state that he should not drive and suggest that he is safer in a structured environment but stop short of stating that he cannot live on his own. He is very angry at his daughter who placed him here, believing that she is "after his money." Your interviews with her and observations of her visits over the past 3 months leave you convinced that she is trying to do the right thing for her father. She has stood by him through three hospitalizations in 2 years that were directly or indirectly caused by his inconsistent self-care when living in an apartment. She is stretched too thin to provide daily care for him in an apartment because of the demands of her job and children. If he moves to an apartment, she will inevitably be engaged in picking up the pieces after each health crisis. She agonizes over his misery and wants to support his move to an apartment, but she is afraid of the next crisis that will disrupt her life and be a risk to his.

recipient. Care recipients often lose control over basic aspects of their body care and environment.

The surprise we experience as family members enter and exit our lives, and develop and lose skills and abilities, occurs because families live in a life event web (Pruchno, Blow, & Smyer, 1984). An impact on one part of the web reverberates throughout the web. Adolescents feel the effects of their parents' divorce and so do their grandparents. A chronically ill child fully reshapes the life structure of the parents and often the grandparents. Alzheimer's disease in an elderly person has a ripple effect throughout the web of family connections. Changes in care needs create major waves across the web.

Caring for another adult family member inevitably affects basic family patterns of nurturance, communication, roles, power, and time structures (Rolland, 1994). Previous patterns of giving and receiving nurturance are disrupted as the balance of caregiving tips in one direction. When the scale tips fully, and one person relies totally on another, new issues arise. How is the care recipient going to nurture the caregiver in return? How does the care recipient communicate anger safely toward the caregiver on whom he relies for everything? How does the caregiver balance power in the relationship? How do caregivers create time for "self" in the midst of caring responsibilities, a common dyadic challenge that becomes more complicated when members of the dyad are in roles of caregiver and care recipient? How do care recipients control basic aspects of their daily schedule without constraining the caregiver's activity choices? Families experience transitions in the patterns of behavior in basic life domains as members age, just as they do at many other points in the family life cycle.

Among the more challenging aspects of caregiving is the range of decisions one makes with and for another person. Decisions that a cognitively impaired husband once made without even informing his wife are now sitting on her decision-making plate. What to wear today? What to choose for lunch? When to go to bed? Whether to bathe today or tomorrow? Assuming that the husband is cooperative and appreciative of decision-making assistance, the load is still daunting.

Caregivers make daily and hourly decisions about how to accomplish activities of daily living (ADLs). The decisions become more complicated when the care recipient does not understand the scope or consequences of various decisions. For example, a care recipient with severe memory problems who always protests at bath time may have no sense of how many days have passed since the last bath. The caregiver then must decide whether the bath is truly needed today and how best to broach the topic to generate the least distress for both of them.

Weightier decisions also occur with unusual frequency for caregivers. Which health insurance plan provides the best coverage for the care recipient's particular medications, pattern of physician visits to specialists versus primary care, and recent health history? Which long-term-care insurance plan covers the services most likely to be needed by someone with these illnesses or disabilities? How safe is she in her own home? Is the house adequately outfitted with safety features? How and when will it work for the caregiver to discuss end-of-life care options with the care recipient? What are the costs versus benefits of taking a new medication to prevent a particular disease? The list seems endless to the caregiver faced with full responsibility for another person's well-being.

Although we watch the generations ahead of us age and care for those older than them, we are still surprised by the experience of caring for our own elderly family members. Both the practical aspects of care and the emotional experience of caring are uncharted territory until we experience them firsthand.

Caregiving on Top of Everything Else

Caring for family is rarely the only demand in one's life. Midlife adults encounter elder care at a time of exceptional role engagement, perhaps a time of overload. Even spousal caregivers who no longer have work or in-home parenting roles have multiple other roles as friend, volunteer, worker, mother, grandmother, and so on, that are affected by caregiving responsibilities. Caregiving responsibilities for a frail older adult sit on top of everything else that makes up a full, busy life.

The research on caregivers' role overload paints a more complex picture than a simple additive or geometric addition of caregiving burden; however, Stephens and Franks (2009) documented that working caregivers with high job satisfaction do better when working than when focusing solely on caregiving. Multiple roles are not inevitably problematic. However, lower job satisfaction combined with caregiving can leave the person feeling the strains of being pulled in multiple directions.

Caregivers do not work alone in most families, adding new dimensions to family dynamics that are sufficiently complicated in most families without the overlay of caregiving challenges and role changes. Indeed, 66% of caregivers report that at least one other person helps the care recipient, although among spousal caregivers that percentage drops substantially (National Alliance for Caregiving, 2009). The primary caregiver may carry most of the load, but he or she relies on others for assistance, support, and input on decisions. Conversations, e-mails, visits, and other forms of communication that caregiving family members use to process the caregiving situation have been in use for other purposes within the family as well. In other words, family dynamics existed long before the caregiving situation arose and are the context within which all caregiving transactions occur.

Communications about caregiving often have multiple layers of meaning for the participants. Consider the communication flow when a caregiver observes a change in the care recipient. The observer is likely to check out her observation with at least one other person, revisit the care recipient to see if the change has been stable, and then contact others to collaborate on what to do next. Each person who receives a call from the observer may choose to contact the care recipient to check out the problem directly and then call to confer with others. Each person may also tell someone else, and so on. In other words, information flows through a family in reverberating pathways rather than in linear sequences. The current information flow likely follows long-term communication pathways, laid down over years. The image in Figure 1.2 depicts the circularity and complexity of family communication sequences.

As depicted in Figure 1.2, the primary caregiver is a daughter who observes something in her mother that worries her. She calls her own daughter and sister to find out if they have witnessed the same behavior, after which each of them calls Grandma directly to check for themselves. They also each call back to the primary caregiver to report their updated observation, and the sister calls an ex-sister-in-law who is still close to Grandma. After checking in for herself, the ex-sister-in-law

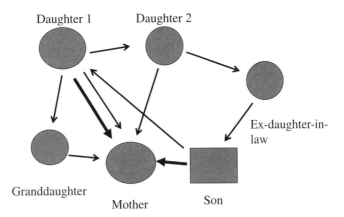

FIGURE 1.2

Daughter 1   Daughter 2

Ex-daughter-in-law

Granddaughter

Mother   Son

Family communication is circular and multidirectional.

enjoys calling her ex-husband, the caregiver's brother, to share the news for the first time that the family is concerned about his mother. Annoyed to be hearing this from his ex-wife, he makes a cursory call to his mother to see whether there really is an issue and then calls his sister to chide her for making a big deal out of nothing because their mother denied having any problem at all.

Myriad complicated, layered scenarios are played out every day in families everywhere because caregiving arrives in families with ongoing complex structures and dynamics. Caregivers who must make decisions about how to interpret small changes (are they symptoms?) often include other family members as collateral sources of information. The reverberations proceed from there along well-established pathways of communication that embody the alliances and conflicts within the family. Truly, caregiving communication happens on top of, in the middle of, and underneath everything else.

When and How Do Families Become Caregivers?

Family relationships are dominated by reciprocal caring actions, feelings, and affirmations throughout the life span (Carter & McGoldrick, 1989; Fingerman, Miller, & Seidel, 2009). National surveys of caregivers have defined the role as "unpaid care to a relative or friend . . . to help them take care of themselves. Unpaid care may include help with personal needs or household chores" (National Alliance for Caregiving, 2009, p. 2). Within families, *caregiving* is the term used to describe a long-term shift that tips the reciprocity balance in one direction, toward overbenefitting one member at one particular moment in time. Parenting children has been the prototype for caregiving over long periods; short-term caregiving examples include care for a spouse, child, or friend after surgery or during a bout of flu. Within families, members change roles often, shifting who plays the roles of caregiver and care recipient multiple times over the life span. At the light end of caregiving, a family member may be mowing the lawn or assisting with complex financial management, whereas at the heavier end of the load there is nonstop oversight of day-to-day life. Indeed, there exists no gold standard for the amount of time a person must spend caring for another person in order to be labeled *caregiver* (as opposed to simply a caring family member), but the consistent theme is that caregivers provide services that assist a person in daily life tasks beyond what is done reciprocally between mutual adults.

Family members often wait to call themselves *caregivers* until they have become quite involved, providing several hours of services each week for an older adult family member. The tipping point is not always evident, even to the family itself. In large part, the ambiguity is grounded in the family's definition of family care. One family may include cleaning house, cooking, and writing out bills as a part of normal reciprocity, without engaging the term *caregiver* even when, for example, a daughter provides far more assistance to her mother than vice versa. Another family labels any assistance as a *caregiving activity* (e.g., mowing a lawn), reflecting their typical pattern of limiting family involvement to social contact that involves no reciprocal services. Yet other families enable multiple persons with disabilities to retain maximal independence by engaging in reciprocal caregiving. At the most general level, *caregiver* refers to a person who provides significant oversight and/or work for another person. In other words, in addition to the work involved in his or her own life, a caregiver takes some of the responsibility and does some of the work for the life of another person.

The processes by which family members transition into the role of caregiver vary substantially, shaped by the circumstances surrounding onset of the care recipients' illnesses and disabilities. Family members may become caregivers when a major illness or accident undermines the previous good health of a person. Sudden, unexpected onsets such as occur with a stroke, propel family members into caregiving roles immediately. In contrast, Parkinson's disease, kidney disease, and dementias such as Alzheimer's disease provoke a slow transition that may be marked by critical events, yet the general trajectory is defined by insidious, persistent decline over a long period of time. Some caregivers have experienced the role throughout their lives as they always contributed to the care of a parent, child, or sibling.

Where and How Do Caregiving Families Seek Help?

Researchers actually know little about how families decide to seek help for care recipients or for themselves. Anecdotal data abound with descriptions of a parent who hasn't seen a doctor in 30 years and had a fourth car accident before family members insisted on evaluation. We hear constant complaints from families about how hard it is to find the services they need when they need them. We also hear caregiver service providers express frustration that families will not access information sessions or classes until they are in a crisis. Families facing aging care needs are similar to families at all other stages of the life cycle: They seek information for the life stage they are in only when they need it, rarely accessing information about what lies ahead developmentally for their loved ones. Not surprisingly, when we first respond to changes in our loved ones, we are often confused by what is happening within them and wonder how to provide help or find services that could be useful.

We do know that most families dealing with illnesses with insidious onset, such as dementias, delay a long time in seeking services (Knopman, Donohue, & Gutterman, 2000) and even in identifying themselves as caregivers (Nichols & Martindale-Adams, 2006). Despite the fact that early detection of diseases is a major public health goal, families are simply not figuring out how to get answers to early concerns. For example, families of older adults with dementia tell us that they recognized changes years before they resolved to seek assistance and then delayed accessing those services for about a year (Knopman et al., 2000). While they wait, their older family members decline in function with increasing risks to safety and independence.

Illnesses and disabilities with more sudden onset often involve acute medical care for some period after which families are expected to take over the chronic care. Family involvement during the acute crisis is tinged with anxiety about risks and outcomes, confusion about complex medical interventions, and disrupted routines to be at the hospital. The discharge process from hospitals is often stressful, with unpredictable timing of discharge and considerable work to obtain equipment or supplies and medications needed for the transition home that must be done in urgent, short time frames. Thus, the chronic caregiving period begins in a flurry of urgent activity with little guidance or even time to think about the long-term adjustments facing the family.

Unfortunately, service systems have not made it easy for families to gain support, information, or guidance during the transition to, or implementation of, the caregiving phase of the family life cycle. Health information about a loved one may be available from a primary care provider if the family member insists on accompanying the older person into the examination room. Resource information is available from Area Agencies on Aging about local resources if you ask for exactly what you need—which, of course, presumes that you know what you need. Families like Linda's (see Chapter 8) are not ready to seek information about specific resources. They simply want to know whether to be worried, when they need to step in, and how to deal with their mother who insists that she has no problem and needs no help. They want guidance as they walk through the ambiguous situation facing them.

We have noticed that some families seek assistance in our clinic very early in an older adult's illness trajectory, at a time when the family is primarily confused and worried about changes that are beginning. The primary factor driving early help seeking may be a vague concern that is tempered by the fear that they are being silly to worry so soon. Such families may be monitoring an older adult family member, perhaps checking out voice tone as a sign of health when speaking on the phone or checking the range and adequacy of diet or the state of the house and yard upkeep. On the other hand, a worried person may be bathing her mother several times per week, managing finances and an appointment calendar, but still not self-identify as a caregiver. Spouses often adapt gradually to illness in their partners so that, like the metaphorical frog in the pot of water, the heat has increased to the point of a boil without anyone being aware of the impending trauma.

The Caregiver Journey as an Adaptation to Progressive Care Needs

The work of CFT is remarkably varied because of characteristics of the care recipient's illness or disability trajectory and the processes that need to be implemented to move the family along toward more effective caregiving (see the example in Exhibit 1.2). As is discussed in more detail in Chapter 2, obtaining a clear picture of the care recipient may not be a simple process. However, locating the family's position along the caregiving journey is a key starting point for CFT.

EXHIBIT 1.2

Dr. Moon

In one afternoon of appointments, therapist Dr. Moon will find caregiver family therapy (CFT) useful with quite different families. The Alvarez family session involves a daughter and son-in-law who have asked for help getting her mother to quit yelling at her father who "just seems so depressed." Next, Dr. Moon meets with Mrs. Glass to help her figure out how often she should visit her husband in the memory care unit to which he just moved; she hates to go and yet can't leave once there because he always demands to come home. Later, two sisters from the Shin family begin working through their decades-long conflict that now is interfering with their mother's care so dramatically that her skilled nursing facility successfully petitioned the court for a review of guardianship; the court is requiring the daughters to complete therapy as a condition for maintaining guardianship.

Dr. Moon's three client families are at very different stages in the caregiving journey and not surprisingly have different concerns and needs. Dr. Moon will want to consider many factors in designing her intervention, including the family role of each client (daughter and son-in-law, wife, daughters), the understanding that the family has of the care recipient's needs and care environment, and the caregiver's immediate level of distress. Obviously, the family structure and dynamics, along with cultural contexts (e.g., racial and ethnic identity, immigration/acculturation status, social class and other resources, religion and values) are also major factors that influence the ways in which CFT therapists work. As a beginning point, however, Dr. Moon needs to fully understand each care recipient's actual illness and disability trajectory, including current needs and how those are met.

THE YOKED LIVES OF CAREGIVER AND CARE RECIPIENT

Similar to the families with whom Dr. Moon met (in Exhibit 1.2), most families walk a long journey as a family prior to any caregiving activity related to an older adult. Family journeys are filled with shifting relationships that Minuchin (1974) referred to as a "family kaleidoscope," within which a small change in position generated a very different image from the same pieces of glass. Family members' lives are yoked in meaning such that even efforts to sever ties cannot be a single person's experience because a cutoff relationship between two people has meaning for many. Thus, changes in the well-being or functioning of an older person inevitably have meaning and impact on other family members.

The years during which families provide care for older family members witness significant change in caregiving services and relationships over time, primarily because of the shifts in the functioning of the older person that are caused by deteriorating chronic disease. Some scholars use a career metaphor to describe the transitions over time, as caregivers must gain skills and knowledge and shift attitudes to accompany various role transitions over time (Aneshensel, Pearlin, Mullan, Zarit, &

Whitlatch, 1995). Another metaphor of caregiving as journey illustrates how caregiving is a series of experiences along a pathway that takes families to places they had not imagined. Together, these powerful metaphors capture many of the ways in which families have described their surprise at unexpected "turns in the road," the steep learning curve for the many role transitions, and the experience of gaining maturity—or burning out—as a result of having provided care to an older adult.

CFT presumes that the developmental processes of the older adult who is receiving care and the person(s) providing care are inevitably yoked. The older adult's process is often characterized by a downward trajectory of overall health, with periods of respite from the decline and sometimes periods of recovery of previous function. Even chronic illnesses have periods of stability and gain that punctuate other phases of decline. Over long periods of time, loss outpaces gain, but the short view may bring into focus gain, loss, or stability. Furthermore, older adults are not engaged in a single trajectory of gain and loss but have multiple trajectories overlapping at a given moment in time. Just as multiple organ systems in the body can have varied statuses of health or illness, so can overall functional status vary across functional domains (e.g., mobility, cognitive functioning, social engagement). As has been noted for decades by life-span psychologists, development is multidirectional, multidimensional, and a mix of gains and losses (Baltes, Lindenberger, & Staudinger, 2006). Any effort to specify invariant phases of a journey inevitably runs counter to the realities of human variability. Yet seasoned clinicians use signs as indicators of more complex factors that should be monitored.

BENEFICENCE VERSUS AUTONOMY

Caregivers need to mirror developmental changes in the care recipient with responsive shifts in the family's involvement. Across the life span, families seek to balance the values of beneficence and autonomy as they support members. Parents of young children ease their way from full legal and ethical responsibility for their children's well-being to the point at which, by middle adulthood, the children are fully mutually autonomous with their parents. The process is fraught with ambiguity and nearly constant transition during the phase of child development, requiring parents to be aware of the child's shifting needs and, ideally, to apply a developmental frame to the psychosocial as well as biological growth prompting those changing needs. Placed within a developmental frame, parents have a chance to view the child's changes as illustrative of developmental growth.

In later life, losses due to chronic illness or disability leave families with the task of figuring out how to fill in gaps in function that emerge. The dance in later life engages the family in following the lead of the older adult, often on a day-to-day or moment-to-moment basis. Shifting from full mutual autonomy toward increasing responsibility, families must shift their support strategies to incorporate more intrusive strategies that would be highly offensive between mutually attentive adults. Meanwhile, many care recipients continue to give back to caregivers in substantive ways, through love and caring, gratitude, forgiveness, funding, and so on.

Stages of Family Caregiving

Although each family's journey into older adult caregiving occurs in a unique, particular context, conceptualizing this journey as a series of loosely defined stages can offer useful signposts to families and those helping them navigate unknown territory. Families experiencing sudden onset illness or disability may jump across several stages if the care recipient's functioning changes dramatically, and recovery from an acute debilitating illness may allow families to move back to previous stages. The key value of this staging concept is that it helps families identify the roles they need to fulfill while a loved one's functioning is at a particular level.

Older adult caregiving can be conceptualized as one form of a normal family process. In other words, families are always caregivers, even though the form and intensity of caring behavior varies according to the perceived functional needs of the recipient. Perhaps the most obvious example is the way parents alter their caring behavior to nurture development of children as they progress through childhood and adolescence. Less obvious are the adaptations to caring behaviors during the period now called *emerging adulthood* (Arnett, 2004), when parents' caring behaviors continue to predict future well-being of their adult children (Aquilino, 2006). Caregiving happens at other points in the life span as well. For example, family members change their care patterns during a period when adults cope with traumas, divorce, and other life transitions or with extraordinary demands such as caring for a child with profound disability.

Just as families move up and down the caregiving continuum with children, adolescents, and emerging adults, adult caregivers also must alter their style of providing care as a member's capacity for self-regulation and autonomy changes. Adults face the same ambiguity in determining when and how to alter caring behavior toward an older person that parents experience during child rearing. Variations in functioning across days or hours because of illness, medications, or diurnal variation in brain function all create a need for change in caregiver services. Indeed, functional changes are often subtle, domain specific, and of confusing etiology. Observers are not sure if social withdrawal is a choice to spend time reflecting or is caused by depression that can only be improved if the person has social contact that needs to be encouraged or structured by loving family. If this sounds tricky, it should. Even the best of parents and caregivers of children struggle with the shifting roles accompanied by confusing emotions and shifting frameworks.

Despite the variability in functioning that can, and does, occur over time and across domains, chronic illness trajectories follow a general pathway from full functioning prior to onset of illness toward death that is characterized by loss of higher level function prior to more basic functioning. Acute exacerbations and sudden unexpected major health crises do not fit the general rule, of course, leading to a nearly infinite variety of pathways that an illness can take. The journey can be mapped in very general terms as occurring within stages that are defined by the care recipient's functional abilities and the reciprocal needs for care by family. Pfeiffer (1999) outlined such a series of stages for families dealing with dementia, for example. Other illnesses and conditions can be similarly mapped as trajectories (Gabriel, 2011).

We conceptualize the journey as proceeding through the following stages as depicted in Figure 1.3: precaregiving, transition to caring, early caregiving, middle caregiving, late caregiving, and older adult death. Although viewing the full continuum as a journey is appropriate for chronic disease, as previously noted, acute illness can move a family from precaregiving to any other stage in a single jump if functioning is interrupted dramatically by an acute illness or disability.

FIGURE 1.3

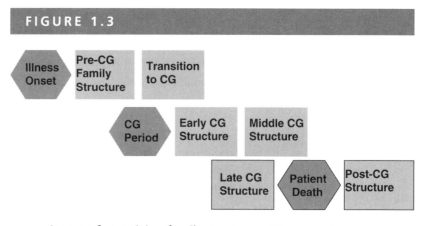

Stages of caregiving family structures. CG = caregiver.

PRECAREGIVING

Family members may only recognize their movement along the caring continuum into a caregiving journey in retrospect. Dementia caregivers, for example, recognize that the signs and symptoms were present in the patient long before anyone acknowledged it or even considered seeking medical evaluation (Knopman et al., 2000). Slow loss of visual functioning from macular degeneration or growing immobility from deteriorating vertebrae are also likely to elicit family involvement in care behaviors gradually. Looking back, family members can more accurately label the points at which subtle changes in functioning signaled a need for assistance. At the time, however, the family is struggling with whether there is a problem and, if so, how worried they should they be and how much work they should do.

Despite their uncertainty, family members often are distressed at changes in the older family member. A very wide range of observations evoke concern: slower physical mobility, visible responses to pain, forgotten details, reduced activity schedules, social withdrawal, unprovoked anger, daytime sleepiness, tremor, shortness of breath . . . the list is almost endless. We actually have data on family retrospective descriptions of early dementia symptoms (Knopman et al., 2000), but the range of possible behavioral changes that elicit concern is much broader, of course, encompassing all aspects of physical, psychological, and social functioning.

Health psychologists have tracked the processes by which we interpret physical symptoms in our own bodies to determine when we should seek medical care (Leventhal, Brissette, & Leventhal, 2003), but little research has been done about how we track symptoms in others. Likely, we engage in a somewhat similar process of comparing the observed behavior against our schema for the person as well as our schema for various possible causes. Slow mobility likely would be compared with the person's gait in previous decades and motivational characteristics, such as the perceived urgency of the journey. Beliefs about illness are powerful influencers on how symptoms are interpreted and the actions taken to address them (Rolland, 1994).

Changes in social, emotional, and cognitive behavior that are characteristic of early signs of cognitive impairment can be exceptionally difficult to interpret accurately. Humans have a bias toward interpreting others' negative behaviors as dispositional characteristics, whereas we view our own as caused by factors in the environment (Gilbert & Malone, 1995). Thus, negative cognitive or emotional behaviors offer a wider range of potential attributions that are set against a lifetime of experience, whereas symptoms of physical frailty or dysfunction are likely to elicit hypotheses about physical causes if they represent a stark contrast to past behavior. Impulsive anger that is a common characteristic of early dementias, for example, would automatically elicit an attribution to internal distress or frustration because of personality immaturity or low stress threshold. The observer may be confused by the style of the response as more intensive or immediate, or less inhibited than earlier in life, but continuities with previous experience will also be considered, often fully occurring outside of conscious awareness.

Family members typically begin to change the way they care for older family members by increasing observation, advising, or monitoring long before there is a defined problem. *Filial maturity* (Blenkner, 1965) is the term given to achieving an awareness of one's obligation and ability to provide for family members in need, especially the older generation. Thus, what we call *precaregiving* is really a subtle shift in care that can occur before the balance that is implicit in mutual autonomy begins to tip in one direction. Often no name has been given to the problem yet, and indeed the family is likely confused about the source of the problem in this phase. Assessment of a family member during this phase needs to elucidate in detail the observed problem behavior, the attribution(s) for it, and previous and current efforts to care for the person.

TRANSITION TO CAREGIVING

The recent visibility of the term *caregiver* in the media has helped families recognize that when one member needs chronic help, others become caregivers. The precaregiving stage gives way to caregiving when caring activities are needed to maintain the well-being of another. Caregivers often do not recognize the amount of care they are providing and thus may or may not self-identify as caregivers. Furthermore, there is no gold standard definition of caregiver, so the prevalence of caregiving varies tremendously across research studies because some include anyone who provides a minimum of 4 hours of involvement with an older person each week, whereas others limit the term to persons who do a particular set of tasks.

In the course of the transition to caregiving, family members usually realize there is a definable or diagnosable problem. Sometimes the problem arrives in an acute way, as occurs with stroke or diagnosis of cancer. The majority of problems have a more subtle onset with no discrete moment when everyone acknowledges that the problem has arrived. Caregivers can be frustrated by the day-to-day deficits that are visible because many appear similar to lifelong problems (e.g., depression, laziness or lack of initiation, irritability, blaming others for lost items, anger at not being trusted fully). Even if they do not have an official name for the problem yet, some descriptor is associated with it. The assigned label or name implies characteristics of the problem (or identity), etiology, trajectory, and implied prognosis (Leventhal et al., 2003). Sometimes caregivers ignore the name because they do not understand it or believe it. For example, one highly educated woman described her father as having "dementia, not Alzheimer's or anything like that; just normal aging." Illnesses and disabilities characterized by fluctuations in functioning can be particularly confusing to families. For example, the amount and type of light available affects the functional vision of persons with macular degeneration significantly. The details of a face may be visible one day, and only the outline of the head can be seen the next day. Hearing loss is intensely affected by the acoustics of the environment, so a person who claims not to be able to hear anything in one setting may be able to hear very quiet stimuli in another. Even families with an accurate understanding of a condition are often thrown into confusion by this variation and revert to dispositional attributions to make sense of it.

Regardless of which type of behavior triggers a dispositional attribution, this type of attribution can easily lead family members to blame the care recipient and withdraw assistance, regardless of need. Environmental attributions lead toward action to alter the effects of that adverse situation. Family steps in to read something for the visually impaired person or offers a memory prompt to a person with dementia. Therapists need to listen for phrases such as "she could do it if she wanted to" or "she's so manipulative—I watched her handle it herself yesterday, but today she tells me that I have to help her." Dispositional attributions such as these reduce the probability that a family member will investigate the true functional ability and causes for variations in functional capacity that should guide decisions about what type of caring behavior to offer. Instead, dispositional attributions locate the problem in the person's personality and typically view it as unfixable, leading to frustration, blaming, or withdrawal. Even once they have a name for a condition, families need to be guided into a richer understanding of the variations in function and the environmental contexts that influence functional abilities.

Family observers may be frustrated by the care recipient's response to the problem. The care recipient may be perceived to be magnifying the problem to create excess disability or denying the problem and thus living unsafely. Alzheimer's disease and related dementias bring additional challenges in that the disease itself impairs the patient's ability to recognize the scope or importance of the problem. Although acknowledging that she has a slight memory problem, a prototypical patient will believe that problem has nothing to do with the rest of her life, even in the face of increasing evidence otherwise (e.g., getting lost regularly while driving).

Until this stage, the caregiver and care recipient have been living some version of full mutual autonomy that has its own definition of boundaries around each person's own choices. As such, the precaregiving relationship has established patterns for nurturance, communication, conflict management, and all other aspects of relationship function. Caregiving alters those basic relationship structures, often in profound ways. Early frustrations between caregiver and care recipient often reflect the rubs that occur when old patterns no longer fit well in the new contexts. Adaptation is often implicit, with little explicit conversation about the exact nature of assistance needed and the rules for offering and receiving it. The shift in the balance of care services reverberates through other aspects of the relationship and into other domains of their lives as well. Spousal care recipients often struggle with the shift in the balance of nurturance. Although often unspoken, care recipients frequently question how they can participate in all of the other dimensions of the relationship, given growing dependency for care. In sum, during later life family members continue in the same role structure and dynamics that have characterized their adult–adult relationship while adopting more and more caregiving-related interpersonal patterns, and the proverbial straws are heaping up on the camel.

In families in which the previous version of mutual autonomy was neither full nor shared, this process can become even more challenging because relationships have less flexibility. A daughter whose father doted on her so consistently that she never fully differentiated from him or claimed her personal authority in the relationship has few behavioral options in her repertoire of communications with him. If the trade-off for receiving relentless doting from Dad was that she had to adore him without questioning him, this daughter is unlikely to have ever disagreed with her father, demanded that he take her opinion seriously, or asked him to rely on her for anything previously. Alternatively, a husband who was always in charge of decisions about the couple is frustrated, confused, and helpless when his commands no longer generate compliant behavior in his wife, even though she appears to have fully recovered from the head injury she experienced in a car accident 2 years ago.

During the transition into caregiving, family members on both sides of the caregiving equation (i.e., caregiver and care recipient) attempt to respond to the challenges of the problem. They also both respond to their initial efforts to address it without changing their historical roles. Care is given, but the role definitions remain the same. Families can become increasingly concerned and frustrated with their sense that the world is shifting but without clear signs of exactly where it is going or what they need to be doing about it. Like the rest of us, in the face of solutions that do not work well, they keep trying the same strategy again, with more intensity, until the escalation generates blatantly painful outcomes.

CAREGIVING

The trajectory of caregiving varies tremendously across illnesses. The practical tasks and the emotional transitions are quite different for those caring for a person with Parkinson's disease versus Alzheimer's disease versus stroke versus cancer. The substages of caregiving described in the following subsections were created to organize our understanding of caring for persons with chronic, deteriorating illnesses that also affect cognitive functioning. We believe the overall sequence applies to many chronic illnesses, however, and even can be used to locate the level of adaptation required of the family who is responding to acute illness or crisis. Although continuing to participate in their own care at some level, the care recipients require some assistance with self-care and other practical tasks. The next three stages require adaptation for families dealing with long-term stable caregiving situations such as spinal cord injury that are stable over very long periods or are very short term (e.g., hip replacement) and involve no cognitive impairment.

Early Caregiving

When chronic, deteriorating illnesses or disabilities require older adults to begin to rely on others for assistance, they typically turn to family. Although formal paid care providers may be engaged, seldom does that occur in the early stages. Families pick up most of the tasks needed to sustain maximum independence in the older adult at this phase.

The focus of assistance in the early caregiving phase is on the instrumental activities of daily living (IADLs), typically. IADLs are the daily life tasks that must be accomplished if one is to live independently. Included in the IADLs are shopping, preparing food, managing personal finances, managing appointments and transportation, and housekeeping tasks. (Note the difference between ADLs and IADLs. In contrast to IADLs, ADLs represent more basic, intimate activities to care for the body, such as bathing, dressing, toileting, feeding, ambulating, and transferring. Whereas assistance with IADLs is a harbinger of the onset of caregiving, assistance with ADLs signals a significantly greater level of dependence.) Parenting of adolescents and young adults focuses on preparing them to accomplish IADLs independently. Upon reaching adulthood, most people have integrated these tasks into their lifestyle so fully that they accomplish them automatically without noticing the substantial amount of time and effort involved.

Illnesses and disabilities can undermine the energy and physical or cognitive capabilities to accomplish these tasks independently. Adults who live with chronic disability throughout adulthood find ways to adapt to retain maximum independence in IADL tasks through use of assistive technologies or paid assistance. For adults who are used to being fully independent, however, the loss of ability to accomplish them can represent major threats to independence (see the example in Exhibit 1.3).

Adjustment to diminished capacity to accomplish tasks of daily life requires psychological adjustment, social adjustments, and pragmatic problem solving. Psychologically, we must find a way to receive assistance with dignity, partnering with those who help us to accomplish tasks without humiliation or shame. The social adjustments required during this process are profound because of disruptions in former balances of power, perceived fairness in exchange of assistance, and nurturance give and take. Some problems require investigation of new options for solving new practical problems, such as buttoning a blouse with one hand, tying shoes without bending over, or balancing a checkbook with limited vision.

Among the most challenging adjustments for families are those caused by cognitive impairments due to dementias that impair the older adult's awareness of his or her own capabilities (Orfei, Robinson, Bria, Caltagirone, & Spalletta, 2008). When the older adult cannot recognize the decline, or its scope of impact, family members often feel torn as to how to provide assistance that assures safety while maintaining dignity and maximizing autonomy (see the example in Exhibit 1.4).

The family system adjusts to provide services when any member requires assistance, regardless of age. Members take on new responsibilities that can lead to new roles. The adjustments are sometimes seamless and smooth, requiring no major shifts in basic role structure. Even simple changes can add stress and strain, however.

Although she may not view herself in a new role, a daughter who adds her mother's groceries to the weekly shopping excursion is doing more work—and work that shifts dynamics in the relationship. Indeed, both mother and daughter have adjustments to be made that are sub-

---

EXHIBIT 1.3

Larry

Larry's parkinsonian tremors frustrate him in many daily tasks because he spills things so easily. More and more, he is leaving written correspondence, writing checks for bills, and completion of medical forms to his wife so that others do not have to struggle to read his shaky writing. He really never said anything to her about taking on these tasks, but she just does them, and he is happy to let her. He tries to retain oversight of finances and appointments but increasingly lets her do tasks that might require writing. He finds himself taking a backseat in managing the aspects of the household that were traditionally his.

EXHIBIT 1.4

Abigail

Abigail's children avoid riding in her car if she is driving. None of them will let their children ride with her, and all fear getting a call that she has had a bad accident. But her car is her lifeline to independence. The nearest town is 18 miles away from her small farm, so without a car she is socially isolated and fully dependent on friends or family for every single trip to the doctor, grocery store, church, or Buddy's gravesite. Her family is frozen with fear—afraid to insist that she quit driving and afraid of what will happen if she keeps driving.

stantial. Daughter must carve out more time for shopping and learn her mother's preferences for brands and selections. Mother must learn to state exact preferences when they matter and adjust to using what arrives even if it is not exactly what she had anticipated. Mother gives up freedom to respond spontaneously to in-store sales or unexpected opportunities (raspberries are available this week). Although apparently minor, considerable role change is inherent in this transition of work from one person to another. Not surprisingly, underlying tensions can arise that add stress to each person and strain to the relationship.

Middle Caregiving

Along the trajectory of functional decline, older adults begin to need more comprehensive assistance than the simpler tasks done previously. The same factors in illness decline that lead to deeper involvement in each domain of assistance usually also draw family into helping in more domains of functioning. The daughter who previously helped by buying groceries now may need to make the list and plan the meals, prepare the meals, and monitor the safety of food in the refrigerator. She may need to track food and liquid intake to ensure nutrition and hydration.

Families who begin the caregiving journey with small, isolated task assistance are drawn into more and more comprehensive assistance with a wider array of life tasks. Simple assistance with household tasks involving heavy lifting may progress to more comprehensive assistance with even basic home care tasks if back problems preclude standing for more than a few minutes, or if lung functioning or vision acuity drops low enough. Older adults who need help planning and preparing meals because of cognitive problems likely also will have difficulties that limit their ability to handle personal finances, driving, and medication management. Those with mobility impairments measure the distance they must move to accomplish tasks and make trade-offs with helpers to reduce the demand on their limited energy or strength.

A common family concern during this phase is knowing when it is time to "take over" more tasks. Rarely do we see families who are excessively intrusive in our outpatient clinic setting. In our experience, families more often delay interventions until the danger level is apparent to all, and all efforts to persuade the older adult to engage in safer behavior have failed. The ambiguities of early caregiving family structures become increasingly clear during the middle caregiving phase as new structures become more blatantly necessary. At some point, families gain confidence to move ahead with a decision that may make their older adult loved one angry because the alternative of not taking action leaves the person at intolerably high risk of accident. Families sometimes need outside assistance to see the level of danger they have tolerated, so friends, neighbors, paid care staff, church members, and a host of other interested parties may bring the problem to the family with a clear injunction to act.

The family structures that emerge during this middle caregiving phase involve clearer caregiving roles with stronger sanctions to act on behalf of the older adult. In persons with dementia, families learn to rely less on efforts to persuade the older adult and to develop strategies for bypassing resistance to care that is grounded in the person's inability to see his or her cognitive deficits. These families eventually realize that the older adult can neither join in a reasoned argument of safety risks nor be persuaded to act logically, so family members begin shifting roles. Wives, daughters, and sons become decision makers who inform the older adult what will happen rather than trying to persuade him or her to act. The unspoken previous definitions of *good daughter* or *loving husband* take new shapes. A daughter who previously defined success in her role to involve respect and obedience to her father's wishes must redefine the role to involve decisions that contradict his wishes if that is required to keep him safe from the poor decisions he might make because of Alzheimer's disease.

Families caring for persons with physical impairments and intact cognition struggle differently with the growing need to provide services for a person who is in charge of his or her own care decisions. Care recipients may be demanding of family members, without acknowledgment or even recognition of the impact on other caregiver responsibilities. Alternatively, care recipients may hesitate to request help for fear of imposing, until a crisis makes the need for assistance obvious to family members. Daughters often describe their struggle with saying no to requests for services, reflecting unspoken family rules or internalized meanings about obligation and commitments within families. "She did everything for me when I was a helpless infant; how can I say I don't have time, but I don't!" Spouses end up consumed by the care demands, with no time for their own doctors, dentists, or physical exercise.

As an alternative strategy to handle the escalating care needs, families often figure out that they need to add formal care providers into the caregiving structures during this phase. The level of care needed often requires families to seek paid assistance to supplement what the family can do. The number of hours of care provided exceeds most family members' capacities to provide the services while maintaining other job and family responsibilities. In some circumstances, the care that is needed requires a skill level that exceeds the family's capacity, requiring the hiring of paid, technically skilled staff. Individual providers and entire care systems become part of the care structure as families move through the middle caregiving stage and are increasingly salient in the late caregiving phase. These formal, paid providers function as partners with the family system, at times being incorporated into the system.

Late Caregiving

Older adults who proceed through the full trajectory of decline from chronic disease will eventually require almost complete care assistance. Chronic, deteriorating diseases tend ultimately to render a person essentially immobile and with limited or no communication capability. The care at the end of life requires full bed and body assistance with ADLs. Rarely can one person provide all of the care when the care recipient needs assistance with several ADLs. When these basic self-care abilities are compromised, health care systems describe the person as requiring partial or full assistance. Levels of care (and cost) in assisted living and skilled nursing facilities are determined by the staffing level needed to support ADLs. A spouse who is trying to meet all of the needs of independent living (i.e., IADLs) and handle the personal care ADLs is on a road to significant risk to his or her own well-being. Formal providers almost always need to be involved, either in the home or in a supportive living facility.

As families rely on formal, paid providers in this stage, their caregiving roles shift from hands-on providers to services brokers and advocates. Caring, loving social communication continues but in altered forms as the older person's capabilities to participate in equal, mutual roles diminishes. Families carry the load for maintaining the relationship when the older adult cannot fully share in that responsibility.

End-of-life care has become a specialization within health care and is a specialized phase of family caregiving as well. As the older adult approaches death, families are often confused about when it is time to switch focus from sustaining life to orchestrating quality of life until death. The shift sounds subtle but has profound implications for family role structures. In the early and middle stages of caregiving, families are driven by the question of how to maximize length and quality of life. In

EXHIBIT 1.5

Olivia

Olivia's oncologist told the family that there is only one other drug to try and, frankly, it didn't offer her much chance to survive this cancer. The oncologist described the risks and side effects to her children, who had heard this story repeatedly over the past 7 years. It never occurred to them to ask the oncologist whether this was a reasonable approach; they just heard that there was one more drug, so they presumed they should try it. Olivia's pulmonologist raised the question, however, as to whether the family really wanted to do this. Olivia's lungs simply could not handle one more round of chemotherapy, and the pulmonologist felt obligated to tell them that she was likely to die gasping for air. Olivia was too sedated to be able to participate in the conversation meaningfully. When asked to consult, the psychologist helped the family explore their values about the dying process that they hoped Olivia would have. The culmination of that conversation led the family to an immediate decision to switch from chemotherapy to palliative care. Although her children had been comfortable arranging for her health care, assisted living services, and advanced directives, this decision process seemed different because it addressed core values about life and death. In this new caregiving stage, the decision-making structure shifted, with new members taking the lead as the focus moved from care tasks to advocacy for ending certain services in lieu of a total focus on the quality of life.

late-stage caregiving, families need to begin to also ask how they want to orchestrate death (see the example in Exhibit 1.5).

OLDER ADULT DEATH

When the person with the disability or illness dies, the family structure changes again. Without the care recipient as a focal point, relationships among family members once again are renegotiated. Conversations that have focused on older adult care, often including shared caregiving responsibilities for years, now must seek new common ground. The frequency of contact among involved family members was previously established to handle the demands of caregiving but now must be negotiated on a new basis.

Death brings a new set of caregiving tasks to accomplish also. Immediate practical matters such as planning a funeral or memorial service; removing personal items from an apartment or senior living context; and obtaining death certificates and distributing them to appropriate financial, health, and legal agencies consume the days and weeks following the death. Often, the family structure remains intact during this phase, with the caregivers who were active in previous phases taking on many of these same tasks. However, legal documents specify who has charge of executing the will and may detail responsibilities for other financial or ownership tasks. These specifications can shift the caregiving roles to new family members, requiring negotiations about who controls information or access to property. Once again, families face new challenges internal to their organizational structures and in navigating external organizations and systems.

The absence of the older adult from the family structure can also initiate role shifts as other family members pick up the roles that were vacated on his or her death. A common example is the role of kin keeper, often maintained by an older woman in the family well into advanced old age. Families often do not recognize how much information is transmitted by the older adult, leaving a significant information-sharing gap that can isolate segments of the extended family from each other when her information-conduit function ends. In sum, the trajectory of caregiving is molded by the trajectory of illness and associated disabilities.

Types of Caregiver Intervention

Interventions to assist caregivers have been the focus of intensive clinical and research efforts over the past 30 years, almost all with a focus on reducing caregiver stress or burden. The many approaches to helping caregivers include some that are specific for particular illnesses (e.g., dementias) and specific relationships (e.g., spouses). Reviews and meta-analyses of intervention efficacy have organized the types of interventions into categories: education and information, support groups, psychoeducational skill building, individual psychotherapy/counseling, and multicomponent studies (Coon, Gallagher-Thompson, & Thompson, 2003; Pinquart & Sörensen, 2006; Zarit, 2009). As summarized in these review articles, some categories show very little empirical support for efficacy, including education/information alone, and support group participation. Other categories contain several examples of effective approaches (e.g., psychotherapy/counseling) that all focus on a targeted outcome using specified methods. Serious methodological issues undermined the power of many of these studies to find effects, especially the problems of offering interventions to caregivers who did not have the problem at baseline and assessing outcomes that were not targeted by the intervention (Zarit & Femia, 2008).

Ironically, despite the obvious family context of caregivers and care recipients, very few interventions are structured around the family, focusing instead on the caregiver's individual capability to cope with stress, solve problems, and meet care recipient needs. Mary Mittelman and colleagues at the New York University Alzheimer's Disease Center have shown the impressive benefits of an intervention that included family counseling as one of several components (Mittelman et al., 1993;

Mittelman, Roth, Coon, & Haley, 2004). Their family counseling helps families organize to provide more support to the primary caregiver. Adapted from a family systems intervention for Hispanic adolescents, the Miami site within the multisite Resources and Education for Alzheimer's Caregivers' Health project tested a family intervention designed to increase support of the primary caregiver by other family members (Eisdorfer et al., 2003). This site found benefits of the family intervention on caregiver depression when combined with a conference telephone technology package that supported family communication (Belle et al., 2006).

What Is Unique About CFT?

CFT was developed to address a piece missing or minimized in other interventions designed for caregivers to aging persons: the family as a system. In our experience, families struggle to acknowledge the profound level of need in the care recipient, at least in part because of their particular relationship history. Families often seek help in a crisis moment when a decision is needed or new care structures are being forced on them. No prestructured protocol could address those urgent needs or the unique challenges experienced by each family system in solving what may appear to be simple problems. CFT offers a process to guide therapists to address the needs of caregiver, care recipient, and the family in which they typically are embedded.

The family context of the caregiving work appears highly salient to us. Caregivers in our clinic often seem stuck in systems dilemmas that are resolvable when we approach them systematically and conceptualize them systemically. Family members simply need help to make sense of the problems in front of them, assistance in solving those problems, and help shifting roles between caregivers and care recipients as well as among caregivers. They also need some attention paid to sustainability of long-term caregiving plans. The family context is usually highly salient at each step, whether it is the historical family who established beliefs and norms for care, the current family, or even the future family that the caregiver imagines.

We also saw a need to build a broadly applicable clinical model that is designed to be implemented in clinicians' practices across a variety of settings over the full range of the caregiving journey. Families arrive in acute care, primary care, long-term care, social services, and housing settings with their concerns. Caregivers at all points in the caregiving journey may need assistance. In the development of CFT, we have been guided by the combined goals of creating an intervention model with sufficient breadth to meet the range of needs faced by clinicians in practice, with definable protocols sufficient to guide clinicians in efficient action.

As was the case with most interventions, CFT developed in a particular clinical setting in response to particular case demands. The clinic in which CFT was created, the University of Colorado (CU) Aging Center, was in a strong partnership with a local Area Agency on Aging (AAA) that provides short-term care management, respite services, and an information and assistance call-in line. The social worker and AAA director recognized that many clients who walked into their center lacked basic information that was needed to conduct care planning or were in a complex family dynamic that interfered with implementation. Families often were confused about the older adult care recipient's problem itself, including diagnosis, functional abilities, or care needs. When they were referred to us, we responded to these needs by developing strategies for helping families organize (or obtain) assessment data into cognitive frameworks that guided care. Other caregivers understood the condition but were unable to engage in effective planning and problem solving for a variety of reasons that could likely be addressed in counseling, including caregivers experiencing burnout, stress, family conflict, inability to implement desired changes, depression, risk for caregiver illness, and a plethora of family confusions that undermined good care.

Our clinical team used evidence-based caregiver support strategies to address these problems in the individuals but kept running into resistance for implementation that related to interpersonal dynamics within the family. A wife caregiver refused to take time to walk daily because her husband needed her constantly and no one in the family was available to give her a break. A son was livid at his sister for investigating assisted living facilities "behind everyone's back." A blind care recipient refused to ask her family for help because she was tired of hearing about what a whiner she was. A daughter refused to schedule an evaluation of her father's declining cognition because she knew he would refuse to go. In case after case, we found ourselves in the middle of old family dynamics, relationship patterns, or beliefs developed over decades that constrained current actions in ways that undermined good care for either the care recipient or caregiver, or both. As we worked with these dynamics over time, we realized that we had evolved into a systematic approach to caregiver intervention that was highly flexible, clinically responsive, and respectful of the caregiver and care recipient as components of a larger family system that would influence the strategies that would be possible and be effective.

In sum, CFT was developed to provide a systematic, organizing framework that could guide therapists to address a wide array of needs in caregivers dealing with a diversity of diseases and disabilities, at all stages of the caregiving career, within the context of their unique families.

Theoretical Foundations

The CFT model is grounded in four theoretical frameworks: family development, family systems, medical family therapy, and the bio-psychosocial model of well-being. These theories provide a framework that retains information from the family's history along with a lens that focuses more narrowly on the dynamics surrounding the immediate challenges. *Family development theory* outlines the cyclical structure of a family lineage as it passes through socially structured phases defined by the entry and exit of members through partnering, birth, parenting, and launching as they are experienced cyclically and simultaneously by overlapping generations (Rodgers & White, 1993; Walsh, 2003). The family's developmental history explains automatic reactions, expectations, beliefs about others' capabilities and motives, and role configurations. *Family systems theory* focuses more proximally on the dynamics of interaction that shape the patterns of nurturance, conflict, boundaries, and alliances and bonds as families interact with each other (Minuchin, 1974). Family systems theory explains the cyclical patterns of interaction that facilitate or interfere with immediate functioning. *Medical family therapy* frames the relationship between families and chronic illness (McDaniel, Hepworth, & Doherty, 1992), in which family structures shape responses to chronic illness, and chronic illnesses alter family structures. Finally, the *biopsychosocial model* is the overarching frame for multidimensional well-being in physical, psychological, and social domains of life (Engel, 1980; Frankel, Quill, & McDaniel, 2003).

FAMILY DEVELOPMENT THEORY

We view caregiving families as existing in one moment of a flow within a family life cycle that has profoundly shaped, and been shaped by, the individual developmental pathways of members. The family development framework presumes that the entry and exit of family members provoke shifts in the dynamics of the family (Gerson, 1995). We hypothesize that families who have struggled with those shifts previously in the life cycle are at risk of struggling again when older adult members decline in cognitive or physical capacity sufficiently that their role positions change. As is true for other points of family transition, such as adolescence, older adult care is a time fraught with boundary ambiguity (Boss, Caron, Horbal, & Mortimer, 1990). Compromises in the older adult's cognitive and physical capacities push family members to question whether role changes are needed. No signposts or signals tell families when and how the transitions should occur, yet strong family rules exist to maintain existing structures.

Timing is a powerful characteristic of transitions. Even discrete transitions in the family life cycle (e.g., birth, death, a child's entry into school) involve time as a significant variable in the process, with periods of anticipation and adjustment within each transition. Ambiguous transitions have more fluctuating courses as the transitioning person enters and exits temporarily numerous times before the full structural transition is complete. At another complex period of family development, the launching phase, family and individual challenges are sufficient to recognize this a distinct life phase referred to as *emerging adulthood* (Arnett, 2004). Older adult care transitions may be discrete or gradual but are equally complex. Discrete health events such as a stroke or terminal cancer diagnosis catapult a family into an immediate, permanent transition, but years of transitioning occur when the older adult ages normally or with chronic illness or dementia.

Families view transitions as being either on time or off time, a perspective that shapes how the family handles the developmental transition (Hagestad, 1988). *Off-time* events are startling, often coinciding with other life cycle demands that are viewed as incommensurate with the older adult member's transition. A 28-year-old daughter who recently birthed her first child views the task of placing a parent in a nursing home as more off time than does a 60-year-old daughter of the same older adult parent. Off time has both the quality of being unexpected and potentially unfair and can bring conflicts with other family roles. Although families do not have rigid age-based expectations for life-cycle transitions, they do report structured expectations that are the basis for determining if an event is on time or off time (Settersten & Hagestad, 1996). Off-time events add another level of complexity to coping responses and are associated with greater emotional distress. Family interactions during transitions inevitably include high rates of anxiety, distress, and strong doses of defensive behavior from individual members struggling to cope.

FAMILY SYSTEMS THEORY

Family systems theory (Seaburn, Landau-Stanton, & Horwitz, 1995) focuses on the interconnected, circular, redundant behavior patterns within the family. Family structures are illustrated through behavior sequences whose redundancy allows members to anticipate and respond to each other in relatively predictable ways. In other words, behavior has communication value (Watzlawick, Beavin, & Jackson, 1967). Interactions are observed closely to map the redundant cycles of behavior that define the implicit system operating rules. Behavior sequences enact and embody the dynamics, both illustrating and actually creating roles, alliances, strategies for interpersonal problem solving, nurturance, and other significant family dynamics. One way

CFT therapists go about mapping these interpersonal relationships is by drawing family genograms, a version of a family tree that illustrates key structural and dynamic characteristics. More will be said about genograms in Chapter 4 when the focus is on family role structures. Family systems theorists postulate that therapeutic interventions that interrupt interpersonal behavior sequences open the system to the possibility of novel ways of relating, thus creating change.

CFT draws heavily on family systems theory, with modifications to make it useful with later life families. One example of the needed modifications relates to the assumptions that a therapist can make about the core decision-making subsystem. Systems theory in child-rearing families presumes that clear boundaries are needed between parents and children. In later life families, the assumption that parents are in charge of children is no longer relevant, and there are no clear cultural rules about when and how children should or could be in charge of a parent. Later life families involved in therapy include primarily adults—children are in the wings—where the generational subsystems no longer dictate functional dynamics. Decision-making structures may cross generational boundaries when aging parents involve their adult children in choosing a home or car or in making health decisions. Thus, the core decision-making system for arranging and implementing care is often a component of the therapeutic intervention. In sum, family systems theories can be very useful but require modification to be useful in working with aging families. We hope we offer some of those modifications in this book.

MEDICAL FAMILY THERAPY

The application of family development and family systems theories to families dealing with chronic illnesses and delivered within health care settings has emerged as a specialty area for practice (Doherty & Baird, 1983; McDaniel, Campbell, Hepworth, & Lorenz, 2005; McDaniel, Hepworth, & Doherty, 1992; Rolland, 1994). Family caregiving interventions for older adults have rarely borrowed from this tradition, although aging families are well represented in the frameworks and the cases that offer guidance to clinicians.

Medical family therapy explores the meaning of illness as well as its functional impact on family dynamics (McDaniel, Hepworth, & Doherty, 1997; Rolland, 1994). Meaning may be shaped by the historical experience of the family with illnesses and disabilities or may be shaped by proximal factors in the family system or the health care delivery system.

Health care systems are growing in awareness of the key roles of families in health care. Integrated care models for primary care now seek ways to engage not only a range of providers (e.g., mental health) on site, but also strategies for engaging families in health care partnership. Significant barriers to integrating families into patient-centered care

are often experienced by providers, families, and patients in health care settings. Yet significant progress also has been made in conceptualizing strategies to work through those barriers to create family-oriented primary care (McDaniel, Campbell, Hepworth, & Lorenz, 2005).

BIOPSYCHOSOCIAL MODEL

The biopsychosocial model (Engel, 1980) is an overarching paradigm that points to the interconnectedness of all life domains in the well-being of individuals. The framework is now relatively widely accepted as an aspirational paradigm, yet is challenging to implement in service systems (Frankel, Quill, & McDaniel, 2003). The silos within which health care, housing, and social services typically operate present practical challenges to families who often appreciate the profound interconnectedness of biological, psychological, and social well-being in their loved ones' lives. CFT works within the biopsychosocial paradigm in helping caregivers recognize and address all domains of the care recipients' lives and the need to manage the impact of caregiving in all dimensions of the caregivers' own lives.

INTERSECTIONS

The intersection of these theoretical frameworks (family development, family systems, medical family therapy, and biopsychosocial) with the particular cultural context of each client is what makes each intervention different from the last one. The intersection also offers opportunities to extend CFT applications into settings in which family-oriented integrated care is relatively novel. Families of older adults must coordinate care across the industry silos we take for granted.

Taken together, these frameworks provide a wide-angle lens that crosses multiple generations as well as a zoom lens to hone in on the particular interaction patterns that are creating distress or "stuckness" in resolving a problem. Cookie cutter protocols for helping caregivers cope are not likely to work. The term *inevitable ignorance*, a phrase passed along to us by supervisors long ago, describes a therapist's entry point into a family (or any client, for that matter). As you begin interacting with a help-seeking family member who cares for an older adult, you are inevitably ignorant of the family's membership, its developmental history, and certainly its dynamics. Even with very precise information about the older adult's illness, the caregiving tasks, and the immediate problems and resources, we are inevitably ignorant of this family's opportunity and challenge with caregiving. Until we have mapped the family story, understood the developmental trajectory of the family, experienced the redundant systemic interaction cycles, and explored the meaning of illness in this family, we are truly ignorant of what this particular family needs.

Naming and Framing the Caregiving Problem

2

Families are often confused by the unfamiliar landscape of later life health problems. Caregiver family therapy (CFT) begins by helping families align themselves internally and align with their health care providers on understanding the health status of the care recipient. An accurate understanding of the care recipient's needs is foundational to good problem solving, including the development of a good caregiving structure within the family. Health status includes the understanding about illnesses (diagnosis, etiology, treatments) and current status (strength, balance, mobility, energy) and their functional implications. Misalignment results in ineffective or conflicted care strategies that have negative effects for the care recipient as well as for the family and others providing the care.

This step of CFT is called *naming the problem* because the information key to this step involves both objective assessments of the care recipient and assessment of the various care providers' understandings or frames for those problems (case descriptions of this stage elaborated in Chapter 8). The family's presenting problem contains implicit and explicit

DOI: 10.1037/13943-002
Caregiver Family Therapy: Empowering Families to Meet the Challenges of Aging,
by S. H. Qualls and A. A. Williams

assumptions about the care recipient's health conditions and needs. Therapists need to be alert from the beginning to separate fact from metaphor and ensure that problem-solving strategies and caregiving structures are appropriate to the reality of the care recipient's situation. Thus, priority is given early in CFT to obtaining accurate information about the care recipient's real health and daily functioning status along with the belief structures the family uses to understand and communicate about them. Of course, the therapist is gathering a wide range of information about the entire care structure in the course of assessing the care recipient's health situation; this information is critical to document as a foundation for other steps in the CFT intervention.

Family therapy is a highly active approach to intervention that engages therapists in addressing family functioning from the very beginning, starting with the assessment process. CFT therapists respect the family's need to leave each session feeling like they are leaving with something they can use in practical ways, even after the very first session. Often, initial guidance after the first session focuses on how to obtain more information or tentative suggestions of care strategies that test the family's way of implementing change. This early assistance also functions as a strategy for learning about how the family functions. Obviously, immediate engagement does not obviate the need for conducting as thorough of an assessment as the intervention context will allow. Therapists working in the fast-paced world of primary care will necessarily work differently from those in outpatient private practice settings who can contract for multiple sessions. Regardless of setting and contract between therapist and family, CFT therapists must be cognizant of what they do and do not really know, relegating hypotheses about underlying problems in the care recipient, caregiver, or family functioning to true hypothesis status.

In this chapter, we first explain why it is important to name the problem. Next, we identify the three types of naming errors: missing information on health status, inaccurate understanding of known health conditions, and misunderstanding of the stage of caregiving. We then describe interventions to address each of these errors. Finally, we discuss how to review health assessment findings with the caregiver and other family members.

Why Must Families Name the Problem?

Families typically seek help with a particular problem that contains some type of assessment of health status and functioning. "My mother needs to move to assisted living; how can I get her to move?" "I don't trust my dad's driving, but he will never stop on his own; what are my options?" "My husband is so depressed that he just sits for hours without doing anything." "My sister is insisting that our parents move across country to live near her, but they do not want to leave their home of 40 years." "My wife's cancer is progressing rapidly, but she won't talk about death at all, much to my children's distress." Each of these statements contains an explicit or implicit framework for the problem being presented. Consider the statement, "My mother needs to move to assisted living." The son speaking this phrase has some frame for his mother's functional limitations that leads him to believe his mother's difficulties can only be fixed by altering the level of support in her environment. The listening therapist has no idea what kind of data are being used to lead him to conclude that moving is the necessary intervention. Thus, the therapist needs to begin by understanding the sources of data. Perhaps the mother's physician recommended a move. Or the son observed specific behavior errors, such as a kitchen fire while cooking, that suggested risk. Perhaps she has fallen several times in the past few weeks. A new medical diagnosis may have been assigned that is interpreted by the son as meaning that she should be in assisted living.

Without ignoring the client's language for presenting the problem, the CFT therapist must begin working toward a name for the problem in which the therapist can place confidence. Simultaneously, and in a parallel process, the therapist will gather information about the family's frame for the problem, including an understanding of the extent to which family members share a frame or are in dispute over the frame. Therefore, therapy with the caregiving family begins with three key questions: What is the problem? What does the family believe about the problem? And what does the family believe the care recipient needs at this stage of the problem? In other words, we begin almost all caregiver encounters by identifying what is known about the care recipient's problem(s), including the level of ambiguity versus clarity of the situation, and identifying what the family believes about it.

Three types of naming errors, all of which can be addressed by this step of CFT, are made by families. Caregiving families may be functioning with

- missing information on health status,
- inaccurate understanding of known health conditions, and
- misunderstanding of the stage of caregiving.

In other words, families may not know there is a health problem, may have accurate information about health problems but misunderstand it, or may misunderstand how far along the health problems have progressed.

MISSING INFORMATION ON HEALTH STATUS

Families often seek help with their caregiving role despite the fact that they do not have a firm grip on the care recipient's health and functional status. Often, families have framed the problem as aging in a generic way that did not lead them to seek a more specific causal explanation for problems. The care recipients may also be vague about their problems; many older adults talk about "feeling their age" or note that they have lost energy over time, lost hearing or visual acuity, or gained joint pain and stiffness—both of which commonly are attributed to aging. These "normal changes" with age may not be benign, however. A person could suffer from arthritis, high blood pressure, or dysthymia, and if he or she did not go to regular health care appointments, these health concerns would go undiagnosed and untreated. The situation is even more subtle and can be more serious with cognitive decline. In general, memory changes are believed to be associated with advancing age, and in reality they are, to a degree (American Psychological Association, 2012). But even the experts in the field of cognitive aging do not agree on the exact level of change in memory that constitutes a disease process (Visser & Verhey, 2008). Therefore, the lay public is justifiably confused about changes in cognition that are normal with age and those that signal Alzheimer's disease or vascular dementia, and they are especially unclear about diagnoses like mild cognitive impairment (MCI) and whether MCI will develop into a more advanced dementia.

Given that information about a person's health status may be missing, if the person is not regularly evaluated by a health provider or if a problem has gone undiagnosed by physicians, both older adults and their family members can easily misattribute symptoms of health problems to personality traits, such as lack of effort, or normal aging causes. Consider the following statements: "My aunt keeps getting sick with the flu, but she refuses to go to the doctor to see whether something more serious is going on"; "Mom doesn't have the energy and pep she used to"; "My husband doesn't play tennis with his friends these days, and he has even stopped going to the country club with his friends." In all of these scenarios, a physical, psychological, or cognitive problem could be at play, and it takes exploration by a health team to determine the exact nature of the problems. Furthermore, among multiple family members, one person may attribute problems to the older person "getting older," whereas another person may say, "Mom's always been a martyr. She's just playing it up now because she's afraid of all the kids abandoning her." Differences of opinion among multiple family members can lead to serious disagreements about how to handle difficult situations and hamper problem-solving efforts.

INACCURATE UNDERSTANDING OF
KNOWN HEALTH CONDITIONS

Just as families may lack information, once they have a label for the problems their loved ones are experiencing, they may still misunderstand the implications of the diagnoses. "My father was diagnosed with cancer. Will he recover? What will treatment entail? How long is he likely to live?" "My wife had a stroke 2 months ago. I don't know what to expect now that it is time for her to come home from the rehabilitation hospital. Will she ever be herself again?" These questions may be answered in a multitude of ways as determined by the individual situations in each case. For someone with melanoma or skin cancer, the treatment and prognosis are different from those for someone with prostate, breast, or lung cancer. The same is true for someone who has had a stroke. It depends on where the stroke occurred in the brain, the severity of the stroke, and many other factors.

For families dealing with medical health problems, an inaccurate understanding of the diagnosis can lead to inappropriate plans for treatment, misunderstandings about prognosis, and family conflict when family members disagree about what to do next. Age as well as preexisting conditions can also exacerbate the complexity of understanding a medical diagnosis and planning optimal treatment. Most 60-year-old men, if they have adequate health insurance and are otherwise in good health, would likely seek aggressive treatment for prostate cancer, as would 70-year-olds, 80-year-olds, and some 90-year-olds in good health. Consider an 85-year-old man who has had two strokes and now has moderate cognitive impairment and is being cared for in a memory care facility. Decisions about treatment begin to change at this point, and families have more to consider, such as the suffering caused by surgery and recovery periods, the confusion that might be caused by the pain and hospital stay, etc.

Inaccurate understanding about a diagnosis related to cognitive impairment (e.g., Alzheimer's disease or MCI) can also lead to complications within families about how to intervene and support a family member with this type of problem. Family members of a woman who was recently diagnosed with Alzheimer's disease, for example, may suddenly begin treating her like a child, when in reality she is still able to conduct many of her own affairs. If families perceive the diagnosis as meaning the person is suddenly incapacitated, they may jump in too quickly to help and can exacerbate cognitive decline in their loved ones by denying them opportunities that challenge them to exercise their mental faculties. In other situations, family members may emphasize that the impairment is "mild," not recognizing that the impact on daily life poses significant safety risks. When the family does not know what level of care is needed, they may disagree about support strategies that could be helpful to their family member with Alzheimer's disease. Some may believe that a phone call every day to their mother, who lives alone, is exactly what is needed, whereas others in the family may want to immediately change the living situation to provide more support. Each case must be examined on an individual basis in order to determine the appropriate level of support needed, and having objective data about the type and stage of illness helps families to do this.

MISUNDERSTANDING OF THE STAGE OF CAREGIVING

Chronic problems, which dominate the caregiving experience, proceed through a trajectory of decline (as mirrored in the caregiving stages outlined in Chapter 1 of this volume), yet families sometimes misunderstand their status on that trajectory. Some will prematurely judge themselves to be at the end of the care recipient's life span, whereas others believe the care recipient has barely progressed when significant changes have in fact occurred. Someone who has been suffering from debilitating chronic back pain for 10 years may have different thoughts and feelings about what they are willing to go through to try to address the pain. If they have already been through multiple surgeries and experimental treatments, the person may be emotionally and physically exhausted and may not want to continue searching for relief. Of course, each person is an individual, so the CFT therapist must keep in mind that not every care recipient will exhibit identical thoughts and feelings in response to similar situations. The same is true in cases of cognitive impairment. A CFT therapist who hears that a caregiver's mother was diagnosed with Alzheimer's disease 10 years ago may make some reasonable assumptions about the stage of decline. However, depending on the length of delay before diagnosis, knowing the timing of diagnosis may still have limited meaning. Clarifying the stage of illness in cases of both physical and cognitive problems will help both the therapist and caregiver to make sound decisions when it comes to providing adequate levels of support, making decisions about possible courses of treatment, and thinking about the potential time remaining until the care recipient's death.

The endpoint of this phase of work occurs when the CFT therapist communicates his or her understanding back to the caregiver and to the family as a whole as a means of helping the family come to a shared understanding of the situation. Ideally, the family then begins to form a cohesive unit centered on a unifying problem, and family members work together to meet the needs of the care recipient while keeping in mind the needs of the family as a whole.

Assessing the Care Recipient's Health Status

This section addresses the first naming error: missing information on health status. Often, family members lack adequate assessment data about the care recipient's situation to guide them in their initial foray into helping their loved one. CFT helps the family gather existing evaluation data and arrange for needed evaluations, with the goal of achieving a clear definition of the functioning of the care recipient. Depending on the setting and time allotted to this stage of therapy, the caregiver also describes his or her own response to caregiving and beliefs about the care recipient's functioning. These assessment processes give the therapist an opportunity to evaluate the strategies the family uses to gather a full assessment picture, as well as the content of the material that is gathered.

Basic demographic information about the caregiver and care recipient, such as name, age, and ethnicity, begins to establish the foundation onto which other clinical information will be built. Each caregiver client comes to therapy with a unique background, and knowing these details about the client will often guide the therapist to be sensitive to the economic, ethnic, religious, and other contextual variables that can affect treatment and progress (Crowther & Austin, 2009). An informal assessment is particularly challenging in cases in which someone's sociodemographic context was underresourced throughout life, leading to compounding negative effects of decades of insufficient health care, nutrition, and personally meaningful employment (Glymour & Manly, 2008).

The therapist works with the caregiver to garner a complete picture of the care recipient's care needs, functioning level, and health status as assessed by professionals. In some settings, such as primary care, the care recipient will be present as well. Regardless, the therapist will need information from other sources (e.g., health care providers, family observers). Caregivers typically worry about problems in functioning, so a detailed account of the domains of daily life that are challenging the caregiver must be created.

Two key questions about functional deficits are whether the capacity to perform the task can be improved with either rehabilitative health care or some form of prosthetic and which services could fill the gap. Indeed, families may have filled in those gaps with formal or informal services and will be able to report on their utility and acceptability to the care recipient and caregiver.

A clear understanding of the care recipient's physical, cognitive, and emotional functioning allows the therapist to guide the caregiver in problem solving to meet the exact needs of the care recipient. Families and caregivers may not have an exact diagnosis for their family member's problems; instead, they may describe the problems they see without having sought further clarification regarding the origins of physical, behavioral, and cognitive changes (Qualls & Noecker, 2009). Therefore, a caregiver's lack of clarity regarding changes in the care recipient's functioning may be part of the presenting problem.

Multiple methods are combined to assist the client in painting as complete a picture for the therapist as possible. In many cases, CFT therapists discover that the caregiver is not clear about the cause of changes in the care recipient and so recommend a thorough physical exam along with neuropsychological evaluation (when any indicators of cognitive impairment are present) so that both the therapist and the caregiver can move forward in therapy with an accurate picture of the care recipient's medical diagnoses, cognitive capacity, prognosis, and stage of illness. The following sections describe strategies used in CFT to assess the care recipient's needs and the caregiver's view of the problem.

HEALTH CONDITIONS AND TREATMENTS

Records from health care providers include the list of medical conditions, medications and other treatments, and referrals to specialists. The CFT therapist will almost always need this entire set of information, so he or she will likely request permission from the care recipient or the legally sanctioned decision maker to obtain these records at the time of the intake interview. Some effective strategies for getting records from health care providers include using nurses as communication points rather than the doctor and asking for recent chart notes rather than asking for a new summary to be written. Considering health care providers' busy schedules, providers will have an easier time responding to requests for information when caregivers are sensitive to their limited time.

Therapists cannot help the client name the problem if they lack the full set of information from the virtual team of providers who are involved in what is typically uncoordinated care. A virtual team rarely knows who is on the team, what each member's treatment plan is, or even how to communicate with other members of the team. As guides for family caregivers, CFT therapists know to gather information broadly; to integrate it into a logical conceptualization; and, at times, to inform members of the team that others are involved in care that was previously unrecognized. With the family, the therapist needs to translate the various pieces of information into a coordinated, logical conceptual framework that draws on all aspects of biopsychosocial functioning.

DAILY FUNCTIONING

One way of determining the functioning level of care recipients is to determine what day-to-day activities they are able to accomplish on their own and which daily living skills they need assistance with. For example, knowing that a person does his own budgeting and shopping without any significant problems suggests a fairly high level of functioning. Managing a household budget successfully requires an even higher level of skill. Typically, a person struggling with physical disabilities or health problems will not experience trouble with cognitive functioning, yet that person may struggle with carrying heavy sacks of groceries from the car into the house. If a caregiver details that he or she is managing many household tasks and assisting his or her care recipient with some aspects of personal care, the CFT therapist will want to inquire about the nature of the care recipient's difficulties. Does the caregiver assist with personal care because the care recipient is no longer capable physically to conduct those tasks, or is initiation a problem?

Many forms for assessing activities of daily living (ADLs) are available, including what are referred to commonly as the basic self-care ADLs (bathing, dressing, toileting, transferring, ambulating, feeding) and the instrumental activities of daily living (IADLs) that include the skills needed to live independently in the community (e.g., managing finances, appointments, medications, meal preparation, shopping, transportation). Scales that tap these two categories include the Instrumental Activities of Daily Living Scale (Lawton & Brody, 1969), the Gerontological Society of Assessment of Living Skills and Resources (Williams et al., 1991), and the Extended Activities of Daily Living Scale (Gompertz, Pound, & Ebrahim, 1994). For further review of ADL and IADL scales, see Rehab General Neuro-Musculo Best Practice Team (2004).

HEALTH SELF-CARE BEHAVIOR

The CFT therapist will want to assess whether the care recipient is capable of completing his or her own health-related behaviors. A person with diabetes must manage blood sugar levels, but that is not all. Diabetes management includes making a menu, shopping for and cooking healthy foods, and exercise. Someone who has cancer may need support with housekeeping, cooking meals, and driving to appointments, especially during the week or so after chemotherapy. In essence, the CFT therapist wants to know how much self-care the care recipient can manage and which of these activities are taken care of by the caregiver. Another concern is whether the care recipient is willing to complete health self-care behaviors. When care recipients have the capacity to complete these skills but are unwilling to do so, interventions may need to be centered on teaching the caregiver to maintain appropriate boundaries with the care recipient.

MENTAL HEALTH PROBLEMS

Whether the care recipient has mental health problems also needs to be assessed. Depression, anxiety, loneliness, and substance use may all be present in older adults and may exacerbate health problems. Depression can manifest itself differently in older adults than in younger adults; for instance, anhedonia may be more dominant than sad affect, whereas symptoms of depression in younger adults, such as cognitive difficulties and somatic complaints, are commonly present among non-depressed older adults as a result of normal aging processes (Yesavage et al., 1982–1983).

BEHAVIOR PROBLEMS

Caregivers are likely to report particular behaviors in care recipients that are troubling to the caregiver or family. Some are socially difficult behaviors, whereas others simply impact the care recipient. Poor medication management, sedentary behavior and refusal to stretch tight joints, walking several blocks without using appropriate assistive devices—the list of possible behavior problems is endless. CFT therapists document these carefully, seeking to understand the frequency and intensity of problem behaviors as well as the contexts in which they occur. Inquiries about times when they do not occur are also important to forming hypotheses about factors that prompt or maintain the behaviors.

SOURCE AND RELIABILITY OF DIAGNOSIS

Professionals vary in how they evaluate chronic disease generally and mental disorders including cognitive functioning more specifically. Unfortunately, not all assessments are created equal. Generalist health care providers typically provide a provisional diagnosis of complex health care problems and refer their patients to specialists (e.g., endocrinologists, oncologists) for detailed evaluations and health care treatment planning. Similarly, in cases of cognitive decline, primary care providers may conduct a brief cognitive screening, such as the Mini-Mental State Examination (Folstein, Folstein, & McHugh, 1975), and then refer to a neurologist or neuropsychologist for more in-depth evaluation. Determining that a dementia diagnosis is accurate requires that the behavioral and cognitive tests used in the evaluation are reliable and valid. If an individual already has a diagnosis of dementia or cognitive impairment provided by a health provider, the CFT therapist will want to check the source of data on which the diagnosis was created and consider whether additional information is needed.

OVERCOMING RESISTANCE TO EVALUATION

Caregivers may be reluctant to obtain an evaluation because their care recipient has a long-standing, difficult personality that leads them to resist care generally. Caregivers may continue to allow care recipients to make their own decisions regarding their care, even when it becomes obvious that they are not competent to do so. In these situations, caregivers may make the mistake of asking care recipients if they would like to have an evaluation, which they typically decline. The caregiver fails to realize that the care recipient is placing himself or herself at risk, perhaps when he or she is not aware of the dysfunction or danger. The caregiver also fails to see the discrepancy in this situation; the care recipient is reliant on the caregiver's care, yet the care recipient is treated as being capable of making his or her own decisions beyond his or her capacity to do so. In session, it is necessary to point out these discrepancies to the caregiver.

Key questions to ask the caregiver include the following:

- What would happen to your care recipient without your care?
- Who is responsible for keeping your care recipient healthy and safe?
- Do you trust the care recipient's own judgments?
- Is it in the best interest of your loved one to have an evaluation?

Gentle exploration can help caregivers to realize this incongruity and understand that they need to take control of this situation.

HELPING CAREGIVERS GATHER INFORMATION

Although most caregivers, when presented with the idea of obtaining a health assessment, immediately see the value of doing so, many ask the question, "How exactly will I get my mother/father/spouse to agree to be evaluated?" Conversations between therapists and caregivers about gaining cooperation from the care recipient can be very challenging because they hint at the role changes that will need to be made between the previously "equal" partners in the relationship. Changing role structures will be discussed in much more depth as the second point on the triangle in Chapter 4 of this volume, but this particular situation demonstrates how all the points on the CFT processes triangle interact with one another. In order to assess the situation, sometimes a role change needs to occur in which the care recipient is not offered a choice about whether to participate in the assessment process to accomplish naming the problem (see the example in Exhibit 2.1).

Martha

Martha agreed with her therapist that her husband, George, needed to go through a neuro-psychological assessment to determine whether he was capable of continuing to drive and manage his own medications and their finances. However, George insisted that he did not want to be tested, even though he could acknowledge that his memory was slipping at times. Martha asked her CFT therapist how she could persuade George to go through with the assessment, insisting that he had always been resistant to seeing doctors and therapists. The therapist asked Martha whether she would give George a choice about seeing a physician if she came home one day and found him lying on the floor unconscious. Of course, Martha said that she would immediately call the doctor herself. The therapist then related the possible event of George getting into a serious car accident or taking too many medications at once to the hypothetical situation of George being found unconscious. Martha then saw that she was taking too many risks by letting George choose not to be tested. The therapist offered a suggestion that Martha schedule the neuropsychological evaluation and then tell George that they had the appointment. Martha thought that George would not want to be a "no-show" for an appointment, and she thought that he would probably agree to go if she took this approach.

CFT therapists help to draw the connection among various symptoms, taking seriously even vague complaints and suggesting strategies for obtaining more detailed information about the underlying problem. Therapists may coach family members to be specific about their complaints and requests or may choose to make direct contact with health providers to solicit information directly from potential sources. With regard to cognitive problems in particular, caregivers may be more motivated to insist on an evaluation if the therapist points out that not assessing cognitive impairment can have severe consequences to the care recipient (e.g., getting lost, starting a fire in the kitchen) that are as serious as failing to assess and treat a medical illness.

CHALLENGES UNIQUE TO CARING FOR COGNITIVELY IMPAIRED INDIVIDUALS

Caregivers of individuals with cognitive impairment often face unique challenges in CFT. In particular, in addition to medical health conditions and mental health problems, persons with cognitive impairment, as their conditions progress, become unable to recognize their own impairments and arrange for their own health care assessments. Caregivers in this situation may need particular guidance and explanations provided by the CFT therapist to lead them through the process of obtaining in-depth evaluations of the care recipient's problems when the care recipient cannot collaborate and indeed may resist the suggestion that a problem exists.

Deciding Whether to Include the Care Recipient

When the caregiver sets the first appointment, the scheduler will likely ask something about the problem for which help is requested. Cognitive impairment may not be mentioned or even implied, leaving the CFT therapist to figure it out in the initial sessions. Clients sometimes ask whether to bring the care recipient with cognitive impairment. Informally, and definitely not a hard and fast rule, we have noticed that spouses are more likely to assume that they should include the husband or wife in the interview. Children more often want to talk without the parent present. Either starting point can work fine. If a person with suspected cognitive impairment is in the room, the therapist can observe the caregiver's style of engagement, which can range from completely ignoring the care recipient, talking as if he or she is not in the room, to insisting that the care recipient be the only one to tell about his or her daily function. Depending on the setting, the CFT therapist may also serve as the evaluator of cognitive impairment and thus clearly needs direct interaction and alliance with the care recipient. Family members are highly likely to view daily functioning differently from the person with cognitive impairment, so therapists need to either obtain written input or arrange to have separate time with the caregiver by interviewing each separately. As is described in more detail in Chapter 9 (on pragmatics), caregivers who insist that the care recipient acknowledge the same problems at the same intensity level as the caregiver views them will need to be interrupted at some point to avoid perpetuating what could be verbally abusive to the older adult who simply cannot view his or her deficits accurately.

Gathering Information on Health, Functional Status, and Behavior Problems

The range of information previously outlined is critical in sorting out caregiving challenges for persons with cognitive impairment. What may be different is that the care recipient may be unable to provide any of this information reliably or may provide information that is very different from that provided by loved ones or health providers. A full biopsychosocial assessment requires the therapist and caregiver to work together to gather information about the full range of functioning. A distinct component to this information gathering is the depth of information needed on behavior problems and cognitive functioning.

Recognizing Behavior Problems Associated With Cognitive Impairment

The caregiver may not recognize cognitive impairment, but he or she will likely be able to report the difficult behaviors. The most commonly used self-report measure is the Revised Memory and Behavior Problem Checklist (Teri et al., 1992), on which the caregiver reports the frequency of 64 memory-related, depression, and disruption-behavior problems along with the caregiver's reaction (i.e., the degree to which the behaviors "bother or upset" the caregiver; p. 624). Therapists who work a lot with this population may devise a simpler, shorter version if session time is limited. A particularly useful piece of information is which behavior problems are of relatively recent onset versus lifelong. We find it useful to ask which behaviors are different from behaviors of 10 or 15 years ago to help the family contrast today's picture with lifelong patterns. The 10-year time frame is helpful because slow, gradual changes may not be reported by families in response to a question about recent changes if they have grown accustomed to the differences in their loved ones. In short, therapists need to know which behavior problems emerged recently, which emerged slowly over a course of several years, and which have been lifelong.

Obtaining a Neuropsychological Assessment

In many, but not all, cases, a neuropsychological evaluation can help families gain a clearer understanding of the nature of the care recipient's cognitive functioning. Brief mental status exams or cognitive screens lack the range of evaluation to contribute definitively to diagnosis. Neuropsychological evaluation provides critical information about cognitive functioning in multiple domains, which contributes to diagnosis and details a profile of cognitive strengths and weaknesses that informs the family's efforts to meet the care recipient's needs. These instruments and assessment procedures allow the therapist to gain a clear understanding of the behavior problems encountered by the caregiver on a day-to-day basis and the tasks that the care recipient is and is not able to complete on his or her own. Although lengthy, neuropsychological evaluations result in rich information about cognitive strengths and weaknesses that are critical for caregiver interventions, while contributing key input into the diagnostic workup.

If a referral to neuropsychology is needed, the client should be told exactly what to expect. In most cases, caregivers are familiar with medical evaluations but may never have heard of neuropsychological assessments, which may generate undue anxiety for them. Families may fear how to talk about the process of obtaining these assessments, so we offer them the following explanations and suggestions.

Neuropsychological evaluations are a series of behavioral and cognitive tests given to individuals to measure and assess cognitive functioning. The assessment will provide both quantitative and qualitative data that help neuropsychologists determine if any impairment in an individual's cognitive functioning is present. The tests typically given in neuropsychological assessments assess the following areas: visual and verbal memory, working memory, processing speed, expressive and receptive language abilities, reasoning and problem solving, planning, organization, and motor function. The assessment process may take anywhere from an hour to several hours, depending on the approach of the neuropsychologist and the services available in the local community. They can also include psychological assessment data, including depression, anxiety, and personality inventories to help determine if these issues are affecting cognition. On the basis of clinical observations during the evaluation and test data, neuropsychologists can determine what cognitive abilities are impaired or intact. In addition, in many cases the constellation of an individual's cognitive impairments and intact abilities will provide information for the neuropsychologist to make a clinical diagnosis as to the potential cause of an individual's deficits.

The following is a list of conditions that can deleteriously affect an individual's cognitive functioning and can be diagnosed by a neuropsychological evaluation (for a complete list of physical conditions that interfere with cognition, see Kaye & Grigsby, 2007):

- mild cognitive impairment
- Alzheimer's disease
- frontotemporal dementia
- vascular dementia
- delirium
- substance abuse
  - alcohol-induced persisting dementia
  - Korsakoff's syndrome
- Parkinson's disease
- seizure disorders
- strokes
- head injury
- psychiatric disorders
  - depression
  - anxiety

Each of these conditions affects outcomes differently and necessitates different treatment strategies. These conditions can also be comorbid, especially dementia and depression, further complicating the caregiver's ability to understand the care recipient's illness and needs. It is important that the CFT therapist provide this education about what an evaluation will look like and how it will clarify the problem. Caregivers are frequently in a state of confusion and uncertainty and often will appreciate the straightforward and practical guidance. Diagnostic procedures can be intimidating to clients of many types, so learning enough about them to describe the experience to the caregiver or care recipient can be very helpful.

Diagnosing Cognitive Impairment

The CFT therapist should be aware that delays in the diagnosis of cognitive problems, especially in dementia cases, are common. Many families delay seeking medical help for over a year after first recognizing a problem (Knopman, Donohue, & Gutterman, 2000), and the average time period between family members' initial recognition of dementia symptoms, such as memory loss, in their loved one and diagnosis is 29.7 months (Boise, Morgan, Kaye, & Camicioli, 1999). Caregivers may have an inclination that something is wrong but may be unsure of their own judgment (Boise et al., 1999). Questions CFT therapists can ask when caregivers describe behavior problems that could be caused by cognitive impairment include the following:

- Why do you feel your loved one is behaving this way?
- What do you believe is the cause of these cognitive/behavioral/ personality changes?

Additional reasons for the delay in a diagnosis of dementia include emotional difficulty, problems in the family, and problems with the care recipient's personality (Boise et al., 1999). Caregivers and family members often do not want to face the reality that their loved one may have a serious cognitive problem; it may be easier for them to deny that a problem exists. Key questions to ask the caregiver include the following:

- What emotions are you experiencing in relation to your loved one's problem?
- Does it scare you to think that he or she may be declining?
- What does this mean for him or her?
- What does this mean for you?

Many times CFT therapists can discuss the following points with their caregiving clients to help them weigh the pros and cons of obtaining neuropsychological assessments. Having knowledge about a person's diagnosis and prognosis allows family members time for planning for the future. Early detection of cognitive impairment often leads to a longer state of independence for individuals with cognitive impairment and later placement into an assisted living or skilled nursing facility if that should become necessary. When dementia is diagnosed early enough, individuals often benefit from prescription drugs, such as Aricept or Namenda, which can lead to a slower rate of decline. Also, if there is a strong belief by the caregiver that cognitive difficulties are a result of normal aging or are related to depression, then a neuropsychological evaluation can rule out dementia or other conditions. Caregivers may be fearful of obtaining assessment information, and these are just a few topics for discussion that can help challenge the caregiver's apprehension. Key questions to ask the caregiver include the following:

- Do other family members share your perception of the problem?
- Is your family experiencing conflict or tension related to disagreements about the care recipient's functioning?

Cultural background profoundly affects the worldviews of caregivers and their families. A person's culture influences all aspects of life, including how he or she understands and frames disease processes. Dilworth-Anderson and Gibson (2002) investigated the meanings that four ethnic groups—African, Chinese, Hispanic, and European Americans—assigned to problem behaviors associated with dementia. The meanings that were assigned to a family member's illness were believed to be related to normal aging, disease processes, and/or pressure or strain. The findings revealed that European Americans were more likely to understand the dementia process as a medical illness or disease. Chinese Americans and African Americans frequently defined the illness as a part of the normal or natural aging process. Defining dementia as a product of experiences of pressure, stress, anxiety, trauma, or family problems manifested across all four ethnic groups; however, the understanding of how pressure was related to dementia varied across the groups. Chinese Americans associated dementia with pressures and natural aging, whereas European Americans understood dementia as relating to both pressure and mental and physical disease. Hispanic Americans and African Americans, on the other hand, did not connect pressure or strain to other processes, like disease or normal aging. Some Hispanic and African Americans identified dementia as a result of living a difficult, stressful life. In working with caregiver clients, especially individuals of a different ethnic or cultural background, assume that their understanding of the cause of dementia or cognitive impairment includes medical or disease models as well as cultural models.

Clarifying the Family's Understanding of the Care Recipient's Health Conditions

This section addresses the second naming error: inaccurate understanding of known health conditions. Once an accurate diagnosis has been obtained, the CFT therapist works with the caregiver and other family members to reframe their understanding of the care recipient's behavior and symptoms.

RESPECTING METAPHORS

Families use diverse metaphors (e.g., intellectual, religious, emotional) when describing the health statuses of their care recipients, a diversity that CFT therapists respect. When helping caregivers make sense of the diagnostic information from medical or social service professionals, the therapist works to translate the official diagnoses into those metaphors and to bring the family into a comfortable way of adopting the health care system's language to the extent that will help the family function. If a caregiver describes his wife's difficulties as, "She's communing with the angels and preparing to leave this world for another," the CFT therapist would honor the caregiver's frame for his wife's problems and speak with the caregiver about his wife's journey, mirroring his language back to him. If another caregiver explains his mother's illness in medical terms such as, "Her physician told me that her brain is atrophying, and she has plaques and tangles surrounding her neurons," the CFT therapist might draw a rough picture of what that might look like and then ask the caregiver what he thinks that means in terms of his mother's day-to-day functioning, filling in the blanks when the caregiver is unsure. If the caregiver states that his mother may not be able to do things as quickly as in the past because of the plaques and tangles surrounding the cells in her brain, the CFT therapist would affirm this perception and add that over time certain processes likely will deteriorate altogether given the loss of actual neuronal cells in the brain.

Cultural diversity simply requires the therapist to expand the range of metaphors with which to discuss illness. Although no therapist can know every culture's metaphors, we need to become familiar with metaphors from the populations with which we will work most often. Beyond those groups, we can trust our curiosity to lead us through an inquiry into novel frames. Some examples of diverse ways of framing illness are noted here just to make the point that significant difference in language or metaphor can be integrated into our work if we are open and curious. In the Native American culture, the term *sweetblood* is used to describe diabetes and reflects the use of nonmedicalized names for medical problems. Japanese Americans perceive the causes of dementia in varied ways, including genetics, bad karma, family upbringing, insanity, and/or senility (Hikoyeda, Mukoyama, Liou, & Masterson, 2006). Spending time with the caregiver client from another culture exploring the meaning of the diagnosis to that person can help to prevent misunderstandings that are based on cultural differences in interpreting illnesses and their symptoms. CFT therapists are not invested in changing family members' approaches to, and understanding of, their care recipients' disease processes beyond what is needed to clarify what the care recipient is and is not capable of doing for himself or herself. The CFT therapist's motivation is generally to ensure the safety (and also the maximal autonomy) of the care recipient in light of the difficulties he or she experiences related to health concerns.

NAMING TODAY'S FUNCTIONAL STATUS

The assessment process described previously provides the therapist and caregiver with a picture of the care recipient's current functional status. In general, when a person can complete all of his or her own IADLs and ADLs, he or she does not need a caregiver. Typically, IADLs become compromised before ADLs unless an acute physical impairment event occurs (e.g., after a surgery or a fall). IADLs may become complicated in particular for people struggling with cognitive decline. Planning, initiating, and carrying out complicated tasks, such as planting a garden or cooking a holiday meal, may become more and more difficult for aging adults with cognitive impairment. Some types of illnesses can compromise both physical and cognitive abilities, such as stroke and Parkinson's disease, which illustrates the importance of accurately naming the problem in the initial stages of CFT. Many chronic illnesses compromise energy level or mobility, functionally compromising the person's ability to function independently. Sensory impairments can have a similar restrictive effect. Knowing what a person can and cannot do for himself or herself today helps the CFT therapist and caregiver change the structure of care to meet the current needs of the care recipient, increase support when needed, and also seek interventions to improve daily functioning when it is possible.

WORK TOWARD CHANGING ATTRIBUTIONS

The therapist needs to understand how the caregiver perceives the care recipient's problems. Is the caregiver focused on the care recipient's long-standing personality disorder ("She's always been difficult; she's just getting worse")? Does the caregiver think the care recipient is depressed or physically ill ("He's not been himself since Mom died" or "Since the doctor told him he has diabetes, he hasn't had much interest in his usual activities")? Does the caregiver have specific health information that informs her framework for choosing when and how to offer assistance? Which symptoms are troubling to the caregiver? Care recipients' diagnoses and symptom presentations are as varied as caregivers' attributions for those symptoms, and the therapist needs to understand all dimensions of the caregiver/care recipient dyad as part of the assessment of the problem.

EXHIBIT 2.2

Lois

Lois blew up at Melvin yesterday for putting away dishes from the dishwasher that were dirty. She had asked him to put away the clean dishes from the counter and run the dishwasher. She is furious that he is being passive–aggressive. Even with "some dementia," he is able to put away dishes, surely! So this is obviously an issue he has with her.

Misattribution of problems to character problems and normal aging often leads caregivers to feel stymied as to how to intervene. Thoughts such as, "This is how he's always been; how am I supposed to get him to change?" and misinformation such as, "Don't all older adults go through periods of depression?" can keep caregivers from changing their ways of interacting with their care recipients and from seeing their care recipients as needing increased support. Assessing the needs of the care recipient, therefore, serves to firmly establish the caregiver and care recipient roles as necessary for the care recipient's well-being. From this stage in therapy, the therapist can then guide the caregiver to provide the needed supports or to make sure that someone else is in place to provide those supports.

As CFT therapists work with clients to change basic day-to-day activities in order to increase cooperation from care recipients, the therapist will often also notice a change in the caregiver's attributions for problems. For example, at the beginning of treatment, many caregivers believe that their loved ones with cognitive impairment do things on purpose to irritate them, including asking the same questions repeatedly, forgetting important things such as paying bills, and even burning dinner (see the examples in Exhibits 2.2 and 2.3). Caregivers of older adults with chronic or acute illnesses are subject to making misattributions for their care recipients' mood, energy level on a given day, and general well-being. Spouses and adult children of care recipients have a history as family members, and preexisting interaction patterns and personality conflicts often continue during the caregiving journey.

EXHIBIT 2.3

Charles

When Charles returns from a long day at the office, Mamie has not even made the bed or started dinner. What can be done about her complete lack of willingness to help out? He understands she has congestive heart failure, but she certainly can do a few small tasks! Her chronic complaints of fatigue and swollen ankles do not seem like a good reason to ignore basic household tasks.

Only when the caregiver of the cognitively impaired care recipient real-izes that the new behaviors that the care recipient has developed are part of their disease process and are not intentional will the caregiver learn to approach problem behaviors without becoming as angry or frustrated (see the example in Exhibit 2.4). Similarly, the caregiver of the physically declining care recipient will need to learn the factors that produce fluctuations in pain, energy, and other symptoms, so needs can be tracked from day to day as they fluctuate.

EXHIBIT 2.4

Susan

Susan is an African American woman who is a wife, mother, full-time employee, and a care-giver for her father, Jonathan. She believes that her father has needed some level of care all of his life. After growing up in inner city projects, Jonathan had a difficult time finding work and struggled financially, living paycheck to paycheck. At times during his life, he drank heav-ily and complained bitterly about the unfair hand life had dealt him. Susan's mother cared for Jonathan by managing the household and by being a sounding board for Jonathan, who had always struggled with decision making, planning, and follow-through on work or proj-ects. After Susan's mother died 12 years ago, Susan took over her father's care, and for a time, Jonathan lived with Susan. A few years ago, Susan and her husband decided it would be best for their immediate family if they could find another place for Jonathan to live. Now he has an apartment in a senior living complex. Jonathan did well living on his own for a few years, with Susan checking in on him daily, cleaning, cooking, and shopping for him. Recently, however, Susan has noticed that her father's health is declining to the point that he rarely leaves his bed-room, where he sits in a reclining chair, smokes cigarettes, and watches TV most of the day and night. Susan believes her father has an illness that is restricting his ability to walk around his apartment, but she has not been able to convince her father to go to a physician for a checkup.

Susan has recognized a change in her father's behavior but has not yet been able to iden-tify the nature of the changes. Her father may in fact be suffering from a medical illness, but he could also be in the early stages of Alzheimer's disease, be suffering from depression, or be living his preferred lifestyle in later life. Susan knows his past but still has trouble making sense of his current behavior. She needs to gain a clear understanding of what her father is going through in order to plan and make appropriate decisions for his future care.

Susan, in her first session of CFT, pointed out that her father is either unable or unwill-ing to participate in self-care tasks; he has a lack of drive and energy to engage in enjoyable activities; and he appears lethargic, sad, and hopeless. She further indicated that she takes care of all of her father's instrumental activities of daily living as well as several of his activities of daily living, including helping him transfer from his bed to his chair and assisting him with cleaning up after bouts of incontinence. Her attributions for his problems included normal aging, problems with his personality, and depression, all of which pointed to her lack of infor-mation about her father's illness and stage of decline.

The therapist guided Susan in obtaining further information from a primary care physi-cian and a neuropsychologist about any medical and cognitive problems her father is encoun-tering. Gaining information about diagnosis, in Susan's case, meant learning that her father had had a series of small strokes, leading to his current state of deterioration. When Susan realized that a previously undiagnosed medical condition was the cause of her father's decline in functioning, her schema of her father's needs altered drastically.

If a caregiver receives diagnostic information and continues to inaccurately attribute behavior to the care recipient's intent to be difficult, the clinician and caregiver still have therapeutic work to do to change the caregiver's perceptions of the problem. At times a second family member may be perpetuating the belief that "Mom is up to her usual tricks" in the way he or she interacts with the care recipient and the primary caregiver. When this is the case, it can be very helpful to ask that family member to attend a session of therapy with the primary caregiver to clear up any misunderstandings about the care recipient's true capabilities and level of impairment. In other cases, a long history of family interaction patterns sets the stage for caregivers to experience a great deal of difficulty in viewing the care recipient in a new way. Once caregivers and family members recognize that the care recipient needs support, although it can be difficult at times, most caregivers find creative ways to manage situations to improve the overall functioning and integrity of the care recipient.

The following questions can be helpful when trying to understand the caregiver's reaction to the diagnosis:

- How do you feel this diagnosis will affect your loved one? How will it affect you? How will it affect the family?
- Do you anticipate having to make any changes in order to compensate for your loved one's diagnosis? How do you feel it will affect daily living?
- What are your expectations for the future regarding your loved one's care?
- What emotions are you experiencing as a result of the diagnosis? Anxiety? Sadness? Disbelief?
- How will this information be disseminated to other family members? How will they react? Who will be involved in decisions regarding future care?

Clarifying What Lies Ahead

This section addresses the third naming error: misunderstanding the stage of caregiving. After establishing the current level of functioning and the caregivers' understanding of health problems, a critical next step is to project the likely trajectories of functioning given the objective data obtained during the assessment. In the face of ambiguity about the future, encourage the caregiver to consult with a physician to clarify stages of illnesses. Coaching caregivers and care recipients to obtain accurate information about prognoses and health markers to monitor can be very informative to caregivers. For example, when dealing with kidney disease, how long is it feasible to continue dialysis? What does it mean when the physician instructs the care recipient to increase dialysis from 3 to 5 days a week? How will this affect his or her quality of life? What are the symptoms of kidney disease as opposed to kidney failure, and what are the symptoms that become noticeable at each stage of decline? Knowing answers to these questions can guide families in their decisions about how long to prolong treatment, when to begin considering palliative care, and when they might want to enter into a hospice situation.

In situations involving Parkinson's disease, for example, some care recipients develop cognitive impairment, and others do not. Some experience depression secondary to the Parkinson's disease, and others do not. How would the caregiver know whether cognitive impairment or depression is affecting the care recipient's day-to-day functioning? What are the signs to watch for, and in what cases are treatments recommended? These questions must be addressed on a case-by-case basis by health care providers. Caregivers will be most able to make decisions regarding the care and treatment of their loved ones if they know the actual diagnosis, common symptoms associated with those diagnoses, and symptoms to be on alert for as illnesses progress.

Reviewing the Assessment Findings With the Caregiver

Depending on the therapy setting, the therapist integrates the assessment information into an oral or written report and shares it with the caregiver, other family members, and sometimes other providers. The length and detail in the report will vary significantly across settings. In some therapy contexts, when time is limited, writing a full intake report may not be feasible. In such cases, much of the value of writing an integrated intake report can be maintained by going over the assessment information with the caregiver client verbally during therapy sessions. The key is to know the problem, communicate the nature of the problem with the caregiver in terms that the caregiver can relate to, and identify the stage of the caregiving situation. The therapist and caregiver then will determine together who else needs to be informed about the caregiving situation and identify work that needs to be done to ensure that relevant family members can coordinate their problem-solving efforts on the basis of a shared understanding of the situation, to as great a degree as is possible.

The process of reviewing the assessment findings with the caregiver takes some time. The therapist needs to make sure that the primary caregiver has digested the information, understands it fully, and knows the implications of the medical and cognitive diagnoses. For example, if the diagnosis is Alzheimer's disease, the therapist would want to spend some time with the caregiver discussing the usual course of the disease, the timeline, and the types of supports the person with Alzheimer's disease is likely to need at the progressive stages of the disease. If the diagnosis is Parkinson's disease, the therapist will provide information on the physical disabilities that accompany Parkinson's as it develops and also tell the caregiver that cognitive impairment may accompany the disease during its later stages. On the other hand, if the family is dealing with a cancer diagnosis, the CFT therapist will focus on whether the family understands treatment options, wants to pursue certain types of treatments, what those treatments will mean for the care recipient and family, and how they might anticipate changes in functioning of the care recipient across time. Therapists need to be cautious to explain only what they truly understand, but the value of integrating information across providers into a coherent explanation of daily difficulties is enormous. When specialty information is too technical for the therapist to explain, the therapist can help the caregiver create questions to take back to the provider until the family has a solid understanding.

Rarely can the full picture be absorbed in a single setting. Many people leave an office having heard a key piece of information, or maybe two, after which the rest of the conversation was lost. A follow-up session or two are critical to ensure that the caregiver absorbs as much as possible. Written materials may be particularly helpful to share because they can be reviewed later. Ideally, personalized materials are provided, but even general information pamphlets about diagnostic or functional conditions are useful. The National Institutes of Health (http://www.nih.gov) and the Centers for Disease Control and Prevention (http://www.cdc.gov) produce excellent materials that are helpful to have on hand to share with caregivers at the point of feedback.

Disseminating the Name of the Problem Within the Family

CFT therapists work toward disseminating the name of the problem within the family in order to align family members' understanding of the care recipient's health status and functioning. The therapist needs to determine how broadly to disseminate information within the family and the best method of dissemination. Therapists working in different health settings will inevitably have different contextual factors that affect their therapeutic practices. Third party insurance drives much of what is needed in terms of documentation processes and timelines for therapy. A therapist working in an integrated medical setting will likely have much less time allocated per client than a therapist in private practice. Individuals working in social services and residential or housing settings will have yet a different set of guidelines and constraints on their work with caregivers. Therefore, clinicians will likely tailor their approach to providing feedback documentation to meet the needs of their practice settings.

The caregiver and therapist may want to invite the family as a whole to a therapy session to explain the integrated findings, including results of the detailed evaluations such as neuropsychological testing or technical health information obtained from other providers, along with the functional assessment of problems in ADLs and IADLs. We would argue that, at a minimum, going through the assessment material and information verbally with the caregiver and checking for understanding is essential to the practice of CFT. Beyond that step, disseminating information to multiple family members and providing written interpretations of medical and neuropsychological data can be extremely useful to family members when time permits (for an example, see Qualls, 2007a). Some practical strategies include faxing reports and feedback from the neuropsychologist and medical providers and using a conference call during a therapy session to provide family members who live far away an opportunity to ask questions.

Although it is not possible in every family, when all involved family members have reached a shared understanding, the individual family members are more likely to support one another well and provide an optimal level of care for the care recipient. A shared understanding among the caregiver, other family members, health care providers, and—where possible—the care recipient positions the family to meet the absolute needs of the person without smothering him or her with excessive controls and oversight. For families in which there exists a great deal of contention about what supports the care recipient's needs and how to best go about providing for those needs, bringing family members together for the purpose of learning about the care recipient's condition can help families start over in their approach to caregiving, allowing them to develop a care plan that is based on accurate information about the care recipient's current needs. At this point, families can also begin to strategize about how they will know when further supports are needed and make plans for how transitions will occur in care structures. Families with strong communication among those involved in care decisions may simply need to receive copies of relevant reports, including perhaps a cover letter or abbreviated integrative summary from the CFT therapist explaining how the pieces fit together and the key concerns that family members may want to address together on their own.

To determine whether a caregiving family has successfully named the problem with the care recipient, the following questions should be answered:

- Does the family have a name or diagnosis for their loved one?
- Did a professional conduct a formal and reliable assessment, such as a neuropsychological evaluation, to determine that diagnosis?
- Do the primary caregiver and family understand the diagnosis and prognosis for their loved one?
- Is the family aware of how the diagnosis will affect daily living?

Conclusion

Finding a name for the problem is one of the core processes of CFT because many decisions related to care are based on detailed information about the care recipient's functioning. Families may not have an accurate name for physical health or cognitive problems because of missing information, misunderstanding of the diagnoses, or misunderstanding of the stage of illness. The CFT therapist guides caregivers in obtaining appropriate assessment information in order to guide care structuring for the care recipient. Families share information so that they will be on the same page when making decisions about the care recipient's level of care needs.

Structuring Care 3

amilies face many practical problems in loving and supporting older adults with chronic illness and often have trouble locating someone to help them find solutions. Therapists need to be prepared to assist with very practical problem solving for a wide range of illnesses, disabilities, and care circumstances. Caregiving families need their therapists to have more knowledge and skills in social work and case management than is typical in psychotherapy, or even in many family therapy contexts, because community resources are so often key components of the care structure in families of older adults. Geropsychologists generally need a wide range of skills related to health conditions, health care systems, social systems, and housing contexts. Caregiver family therapy (CFT) therapists' use of a family systems framework helps them work with the family dynamics that add complexity to care challenges and care solutions. This chapter describes how CFT therapists can put their systems framework to work as they help families implement fundamental problem-solving strategies in new contexts (case descriptions of this stage provided in Chapter 8).

DOI: 10.1037/13943-003
Caregiver Family Therapy: Empowering Families to Meet the Challenges of Aging,
by S. H. Qualls and A. A. Williams

Addressing Safety Concerns

Although safety is discussed in greater detail later in this chapter, the topic is important enough to warrant a general discussion here. In optimal situations, the therapist, caregiver, and other family members identify the care recipient's needs and address them before any safety concerns can arise. Families can be very creative in their approaches to changing care structures so that the care recipient continues to have as much independence as is possible. Yet while autonomy is important to most individuals, unsupported independence can lead to unsafe outcomes. A person who cannot manage his or her own medications will need support to complete that task. A person who has burned several meals could benefit from supervision while cooking or simplified instructions for using a microwave as a primary means of cooking. A driver with a few recent fender benders may need a driving assessment to determine whether having a license and a car is safe—not only for the care recipient but also for other drivers and pedestrians. Caregivers often have the unpleasant task of communicating concerns and even demanding changes that must occur for the sake of safety. The therapist can help with this process by role-playing, coaching the caregiver through the conversation, and at times suggesting that someone else (e.g., a family physician or other authority figure or a favored child) deliver the news that the care recipient is not going to want to hear. In this situation, the family relationship can be maintained while the behavior of concern is addressed by an outside care provider.

Once any safety concerns have been addressed, the caregiver must still monitor that the care recipient's needs are being met and learn to anticipate when new supports become necessary. For example, if a person with chronic obstructive pulmonary disease experiences health deterioration over time, his caregiver will likely need to increase communication with the health care provider; monitor oxygen intake to ensure its adequacy; and perhaps increase in-home supports, such as housekeeping and cooking services, to reduce the day-to-day physical demands on the care recipient. In cases of cognitive impairment, a person who can manage microwave cooking today may not be able to continue managing this task as her functioning declines. Adding Meals on Wheels or sharing responsibility with other family members for cooking meals for the care recipient are examples of strategies for changing care structures to meet the care recipient's needs.

Throughout the course of the illness, the person with a progressive cognitive disease, such as Alzheimer's disease or other dementia, will continue to need someone to observe and adjust the environment to meet that person's needs. This usually falls to primary caregivers, who are supported by other family members along with a range of formal and informal care providers. CFT therapists also can help the monitoring process by listening for signals that a higher level of support is emerging and communicating that to the caregiver. The stages of caregiving outlined in Chapter 1 of this volume can be shown to a caregiver as a general description of the journey ahead.

Principles to
Guide Interventions

When the picture becomes clear as to what the older adult care recipient needs from the family, what services the family currently provides, and how roles are structured to offer the care, the therapist and client can map unresolved and emerging care needs onto that picture. The map will readily show gaps. We recognize that therapists are infinitely creative in building interventions for families so rely on stating core values and principles to guide them.

MAXIMIZE THE OLDER ADULT'S INVOLVEMENT

CFT supports the engagement of older members to the fullest extent possible in self-direction of decisions that relate to their own lives, including care decisions. Typically, families also want their older members to engage fully in their own care and make their own decisions. Perhaps the simplest way of honoring someone and protecting dignity is to ensure their full voice in decisions.

Families are most likely to struggle with this principle when an older member appears to be making poor choices. Just as at other points in the life span, families struggle with how involved to become with loved ones who use poor judgment: the chronic alcoholic who sacrifices his family to retain his drinking pattern, the abused spouse who stays in the relationship, and the sister whose impulsive job changes undermine financial stability. Situations like these tug at us, generating a desire to help the person stop a self-defeating or self-injurious behavior pattern. We share information, cajole, persuade, assist with picking up the pieces after a situation falls apart, and so on. And sometimes we come to the conclusion that we simply have to live with another person's choice(s) that seem so wrong. Often, we have tried to persuade the person to shift the overall pattern but have been unsuccessful.

Families also struggle to include the care recipient if he or she appears to be declining in the ability to oversee his or her own life. Older family members are invested in retaining full control over their decisions and lifestyle (of course) and may not see the safety risks that families fear, or they may not view or weigh them similarly. With their focus typically on autonomy, older family members may resist hearing about, or acting on, information related to safety risks. The tug of war is not unlike that of parents of adolescents who have an inherently different view of safety risks from that of the invincible, immortal adolescent. Aging family members may understand the safety risks but simply say that they are a tolerable preference over lower risk congregate living environments.

A challenging case we often encounter in our clinic is that of an older adult whose cognitive impairment renders him or her incapable of seeing risks, and therefore his family does not include him in decision making. Unfortunately, one common characteristic of most dementias and some strokes is *anosognosia* or the inability to recognize the scope or importance of one's cognitive difficulties (Orfei, Robinson, Bria, Caltagirone, & Spalletta, 2008). A common phrase spoken by such a person is, "I have some memory problems, but my family is making way too much out of it. I can still drive just fine." By the time they seek help, families may have already tried unsuccessfully to persuade the older adult to see the risks and voluntarily choose a less risky option (e.g., cease driving voluntarily, accept help with medication or financial management). Or, the process of naming the problem (see Chapter 2) helped the family see the need, and they now attempt such persuasion. Occasionally, the person with cognitive impairment will indeed be able to see the risks involved in his or her preferred choice or will simply cooperate with the family's efforts to persuade him or her to change.

Even in cases of older adults with significant cognitive limitations, this principle of maximizing involvement applies. Unless the person has no means of communicating preferences, his or her input should be obtained and used to guide choices. A self-directed life is a basic human right that applies to persons with declining cognitive ability as it does to all others. Even compromised cognitive function does not remove all capability of self-direction. A key question families need assistance with is exactly how the person can and cannot engage in self-direction. Even persons with quite limited cognitive capacity to organize information about their lives can make statements about their preferences and values that need to be considered in family decisions. The question is how to support involvement that is congruent with abilities. Figure 3.1 offers an image of a gradient of involvement that illustrates the varied ways in which older adults might participate in family decision making. At the bottom of the figure, the larger capacity represented by the widest rectangle includes options for the older adult to collaborate fully in the analysis and decision making as a shared

FIGURE 3.1

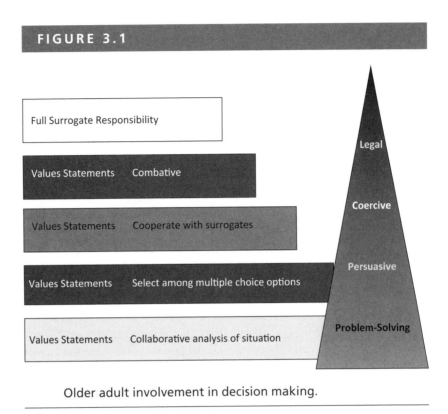

Full Surrogate Responsibility

Values Statements   Combative

Values Statements   Cooperate with surrogates

Values Statements   Select among multiple choice options

Values Statements   Collaborative analysis of situation

Legal

Coercive

Persuasive

Problem-Solving

Older adult involvement in decision making.

problem solver. Moving up the figure, the rectangles become smaller, representing more limited cognitive capacity and styles of collaboration with family that are constrained by those limitations. At almost all levels of cognitive capacity, however, the older person can make values statements. Even when combatively engaged against family choices that are critical to basic safety and well-being, the older person can make a values statement about which residential facility is preferred or which caregiver is preferred.

The principle of maximal involvement guides CFT therapists to seek mechanisms by which older adults can participate and to identify domains in which their preferences and values can be implemented at least partially, if not fully. Often, we guide the family through the process of identifying the contexts in which older adult contributions should be considered (and where they should not be) on the basis of assessment of cognition and functioning. This data-based foundation for deciding where the care recipient's voice can and should be heard is welcomed by families who have wanted to involve the older person but feared being at the mercy of the poor judgment that results from cognitive impairment.

USE THE LEAST INTRUSIVE INTERVENTION THAT ACCOMPLISHES CHANGE

Two models have informed CFT's commitment to this principle. Many therapies share this type of value, including one well-articulated in the field of sex therapy, the PLISSIT model (Annon, 1974). The PLISSIT acronym summarizes four levels of intensity of intervention, ranging from least intrusive to most intensive: permission, limited intervention, specific suggestion, and intensive therapy. The simplicity of this system is applicable to almost all interventions but particularly to those involving interpersonal dynamics. Family members often know what to do but seem to benefit from being given permission to act. When permission is insufficient, a very limited intervention, such as the provision of information about a disease or about others' similar experiences may be sufficient to engage the family in behavior change. Specific suggestions involve a more targeted recommendation, designed specifically for this particular family. "Try saying this . . ." is an example of a specific suggestion. Another example is, "Go ahead and make the appointment with the doctor that your mother needs, and then tell her when it is, rather than waiting for her to make it." Finally, some families require more intensive therapy to restructure their thought or behavior patterns sufficiently to change their roles. Deep grieving of past losses or processing past hurts may be needed before a daughter can engage as a caregiver. Siblings may need to work on their relationship more intensively before being able to collaborate in decision making on behalf of a parent. Simple is often elegant, and we find the PLISSIT model to be a simple, elegant guide for the principle of least intrusive intervention.

Family therapy models often implement this model in their distinction between first-order and second-order change (Watzlawick, Weakland, & Fisch, 1974). *First-order change* involves adaptation of existing structures to address new situations. Therapists can often coach families through a shift in their approach to a problem in order to maximize success in addressing it with approaches such as changing frequency or intensity of communication, shifting reward systems for desired behavior, or adding resources. *Second-order changes* involve a shift in the structure of the family that either renders the problem a nonproblem or opens new possibilities in problem resolution that were not possible in the old structures. For example, a problem with decision making that occurs because of conflict between two people over authority becomes a nonproblem when one person is removed from decision-making authority. Second-order change is inherent in significant family development transitions. Launching a child out of the family home and into a dorm or apartment renders conflicts over at least some aspects of shared domestic life moot (e.g., curfew, room cleanliness). Remarriage of a single parent inevitably alters the decision-making and conflict resolution dynamics between that parent and his or her adolescent child. Transition of a person with dementia to a memory care facility removes him or her from daily financial decisions, potentially leaving the spouse and children to establish new collaborative relationships. New opportunities for addressing problems are now possible because of the new person in the triangle. When familiar patterns are disrupted enough, it is possible for new relationship patterns to emerge. Second-order changes are more intensive than first-order changes, harder to accomplish, and thus typically chosen only when first-order change has not worked.

Each of the two models described previously distinguishes between minor interventions (e.g., permission, limited intervention, and specific suggestions are examples of first-order change) and more substantive interventions (i.e., second-order change and intensive therapy). Caregivers often benefit from relatively minor interventions, but substantial role transitions are also part of the caregiving journey.

BALANCE SAFETY AND AUTONOMY

Development is fraught with risk at all life stages, and families are often caught in a maelstrom of conflict over how to balance the urge toward autonomy with the profound sense of need to protect in order to maintain safety. Optimal developmental pathways in childhood afford options for growing autonomy while offering guidance and nets to maintain safety. Later adulthood makes salient the inevitable tension between safety and autonomy within families again. As the balance of the gains and losses of development tip toward higher rates of losses (Baltes & Baltes, 1990), families often struggle with how to respond. For example,

> Should I offer to help more, or is it good for my mother to have a reason to move around the house more? I certainly don't want her to fall, because the consequences could be devastating to her health. On the other hand, if I keep stepping in to help her, she will lose strength more and more and thus end up losing the option of staying in her own home, which is what she values more than anything.

Just as research on married couples has mapped out the most common sources of marital conflict (e.g., money, child rearing, sex), so later life family therapists can identify common sources of interpersonal conflict within families. The balance of autonomy and safety is one of those areas ripe for conflict, and for good reason.

On the scale balancing safety and autonomy, rarely is there a stable balance point. Rather, the scale tips slightly one way or the other intermittently, occasionally achieving a static moment of perfect balance before shifting slightly again. Fear of experiencing a major tipping point is a challenge for families, leading them to ask questions about when the living circumstances need to be modified to prevent a big tip. Why exactly is she struggling to maintain her home and hygiene? Is she not understanding what is needed, not willing to do it, or not able to do it? Having completed the first phase of CFT (naming the problem), therapist and clients should have a reasonable understanding of the cause, scope, and nature of limitations. Now that it is time to plug in assistance where it is truly needed, the emotional aspects of living with the autonomy–safety balance are salient.

In family systems, some members inevitably have more of a bent toward tracking and ensuring safety, whereas others have a similar bent toward autonomy. Actually, almost all humans appreciate the value of both, but within the family each person may develop a familiar voice that speaks more quickly or passionately about one side of the balance or the other. The source of that preference or style may be personality, or may be more systemic. If one person in a family has a strong voice on one side of the balance, others may naturally drift toward the balancing position and thus become known for that view. A sister who is viewed as cautious may be the natural counterbalance to her older brother's tendency to be a high-risk taker, a voice that was logical in childhood continues in perpetuity. She may instead be a highly anxious person who manages her anxiety through cautious anticipation of even small risks, and thus her voice represents her temperament more than her family position: "She could fall if she walks in the neighborhood every day." Other family members may habitually offer the countervoice: "I'm sure it will be OK for her to try it alone."

Families have the urge to polarize the tension between safety and autonomy between people. Once positioned as an interpersonal problem, rather than as a challenging values dilemma experienced by each person internally (i.e., inherently intraindividual), conflict over care strategies will heat up. Siblings will argue vehemently about the value and appropriateness of a nursing home placement, with one person accusing the other of not caring that Mom has always said she wants to live out her life in her own home, and the other person counteraccusing that the first would be willing to let Mom die alone on a floor just so he or she doesn't have to take responsibility for a hard decision to move Mom (see the example in Exhibit 3.1).

As in many other families, what begins as a very hard question about how to support a person whose declining abilities are putting his or her well-being at risk has deteriorated into a sibling fight whose basic positions have not changed since adolescence. Strategies for dealing with this type of interpersonal implementation of intrapersonal values struggle are outlined next. For now, the point is that the balance between autonomy and safety is inevitably difficult to maintain. Recognizing the inherent tension between the two values is key to figuring out how to help families actively engage in balancing these competing values.

EXHIBIT 3.1

Tom and Janet

When Tom and Janet came into the therapy office, the air in the room was so tense you could cut it with a knife. "What brings you in today?" led to such a torrent of angry interchanges that the therapist had to halt the interaction and provide high levels of structure to keep the conversation from running out of control. Tom claimed that their mother was in mortal danger of food poisoning and medication overdose because she was managing her daily routines so badly. He insisted that it was obvious that she needed to move to a nursing home. Janet angrily countered that moving her to a nursing home would kill her even though it would reduce Tom's responsibilities, which was probably what Tom wanted so he wouldn't have to spend his inheritance taking care of her. Janet stated that she wanted their mother to be able to fulfill her expressed desire to live out her life in the long-term family home. According to Janet, Tom was being overly protective just so he wouldn't have to feel guilty about anything after their mother was gone. Tom's red face exploded in anger that he would be so unjustly accused, and he noted that Janet wanted their mother at home so she could manipulate her to get the money that would otherwise be spent on their mother's care in a nursing home.

A caregiver's functioning, in some ways, can be measured by his or her ability to ensure that all of the care recipient's safety needs are addressed. Decision-making capacity, financial management, risk of exploitation, health care management, medication, nutrition and cooking, falls, driving, and elder abuse are the most frequently encountered safety concerns in CFT. No hard and fast rules exist to guide a caregiver in making decisions about when to step in and provide increased support, but see the section Addressing Specific Concerns in this chapter for some guidelines to assist with thinking about when help is needed. Resources exist in most urban areas to provide assistance for older adults who have needs in these particular areas, whereas a little extra creativity may be necessary to recruit assistance with caregiving in rural areas.

Problem-Solving Model

The stage is set for the therapist and caregiver to work together in structuring care for the care recipient in the process of naming the problem during the first step of CFT (see Chapter 2). The therapist obtained information on the diagnoses and functioning capacity of the care recipient and also identified family member beliefs about and understanding of the diagnosis and care needs of the care recipient. The therapist now begins to ask questions about whether transitions in care and support services are needed, whether the caregiver's role needs to be adjusted to meet the needs of the care recipient, and whether interpersonal negotiations with the care recipient or family members are needed. CFT therapists train caregivers in problem-solving techniques to facilitate changes that may be necessary in the caregiving context. Problem-solving approaches to therapy are used widely by therapists who work with all types of clients. The model we discuss in this chapter will not seem new or novel to most therapists; therefore, we provide only an overview of the model and spend most of the chapter on common problems.

We focus on a model of problem-solving therapy (PST) that has grown out of D'Zurilla and Goldfried's (1971) original paper integrating much of the work that had previously been done on PST. From 1971 until more recently, hundreds of studies have looked at the impact of PST on coping skills, depression, anxiety, and schizophrenia with a variety of clients, including caregivers (for reviews of the literature, see Malouff, Thorsteinsson, & Schutte, 2007; Nezu, 2004). In addition to PST being taught in outpatient mental health settings, researchers have successfully used this approach in long-term-care settings with patients, their families, and staff (Ayalon, Bornfeld, Gum, & Areán, 2008) and in primary care settings with depressed patients (Areán, Hegel, Vannoy, Fan, & Unuzter, 2008). Nezu (2004) pointed out that PST can be one element of a larger treatment package, and that is the way we conceptualize the role of PST in CFT.

PROBLEM-SOLVING APPROACH

D'Zurilla, Nezu, and Maydeu-Olivares (2004) defined *problem solving* as "the process by which people both understand and react to problems in living by altering the problematic nature of the situation itself, the person's reactions to the situation, or both, in their model of social problem solving" (p. 12). This definition is important because it points to the dual focus of problem solving—the focus on the problem itself, as well as on the person who is coping with the problem. According to the PST model, family caregivers who have a positive problem orientation and who use a positive problem-solving style, such as rational problem solving, will be successful. The goals of PST are to increase the caregiver's positive orientation while simultaneously decreasing negative orientation and to improve the caregiver's rational problem-solving skills while decreasing impulsive, careless, and avoidant approaches to problem solving (Nezu, 2004). Nezu, Palmatier, and Nezu (2004) discussed how the PST model is relevant to the caregiver process, and various training programs and interventions for caregivers of chronic illnesses have been developed using the PST model as a guide (i.e., Houts, Nezu, Nezu, & Bucher, 1996; Malouf, Thorsteinsson, & Schutte, 2007; Nezu, 2004; Sahler et al., 2005; Seltzer, Greenberg, & Krauss, 1995). Overall, clients of PST have been found to have less emotional distress and improved psychological functioning (Nezu, 2004).

PROBLEM ORIENTATION

In caregiving for people with chronic physical or cognitive illnesses, *orientation* refers to how the caregiver views his or her role along with the expectations for fulfilling that role successfully. People who approach problems from a positive orientation consider problems as challenges that are ultimately solvable (Nezu, 2004). They also believe in their own ability to solve problems and that doing so requires time and effort (Nezu, 2004). On the other hand, people who are negatively oriented believe that problems are threats and unsolvable. They doubt their own ability to successfully deal with problems and feel frustrated and upset by difficult situations (Nezu, 2004). Overall, *"problem orientation* is the set of relatively stable cognitive affective schemas that represent a person's generalized beliefs, attitudes, and emotional reactions about problems in living and one's ability to successfully cope with such problems" (Nezu, 2004, p. 3). Individuals approaching problems from a positive frame generally experience more positive affect and approach rather than avoid problem solving. On the other hand, individuals with a negative orientation demonstrate poor problem-solving skills and depression, anxiety, and worry, among other psychological and medical problems (Nezu, 2004).

BUILDING SELF-EFFICACY

Caregivers may experience burden, challenge, expectations of failure, and/or a sense of competency in their roles. A positive orientation is extremely important for caregivers and includes the perspective that one's problem-solving efforts, given time and persistence, will be effective. This concept is similar to that of locus of control. A caregiver who believes that he or she has power to make changes in the situation is more likely to formulate solutions and implement them successfully. The therapist may start to enhance this belief by helping the caregiver become more aware of emotional cues as an aid to identifying problems and restructuring cognitive misattributions to difficult situations.

After learning about problem-solving strategies, caregivers should believe that they can tackle most of the day-to-day problems that they will encounter in caregiving for a loved one. The therapist can accomplish this by providing information to the caregiver about how to handle problems commonly associated with the care recipient's condition and by facilitating training on how to be an effective and successful problem solver in dealing with new and often difficult situations.

TEACHING RATIONAL PROBLEM-SOLVING STRATEGIES

Caregivers need to be able to *define the problem* as the first step in the rational problem-solving process, both for themselves and for health professionals overseeing the recipient's care (i.e., nurse, primary care physician, and psychiatrist). Often, that means defining the who, what, and when of the problem as well as how often it occurs. Formulating the problem may involve obtaining expert information from health professionals because the caregiver may have little previous knowledge about the physical and/or cognitive health problems that the care recipient is experiencing. Understanding the diagnosis of the care recipient (see Chapter 2) can help the caregiver and therapist formulate the problem and generate possible solutions.

The second step in rational problem solving is *brainstorming alternatives.* Caregivers who possess a strong ability to generate alternative solutions "are able to maximize the likelihood that the most effective solution will be discovered" (Nezu, Palmatier, & Nezu, 2004, p. 227). When generating alternatives, the caregiver could ask health professionals such as you, the therapist, or a health care provider for ideas or seek information through reading books, searching the Internet, or talking with other people who have experienced similar problems. Support groups are a great place to discover alternative solutions. Often, however, the caregiver is the primary source of creative options, as there may be unique obstacles that he or she is facing. The therapist's job is to help facilitate the generation of possible solutions to some of these challenging situations. Without being disrespectful of the time and investment of the caregiver in the therapy, the client should be encouraged to think outside the box, generating solution options that may seem silly or quite far-fetched initially. Even wild ideas can sometimes be implemented or may point the caregiver to another option that would not have been considered without the "outside the box" moment. In short, the caregiver and therapist should arrive at as many solutions as possible.

Training individuals to make effective decisions involves teaching them to *weigh the pros and cons of each possible solution,* which is the third step in rational problem solving (Nezu, Palmatier, & Nezu, 2004). This includes an evaluation of the likelihood that the solution will be effective and that it will yield the desired consequences for both the care recipient and caregiver. Considering the pros and cons of each option for the caregiver as well as the care recipient is an important skill for the caregiver to learn. Frequently, caregivers make decisions solely based on the needs of the care recipient. This lack of consideration for themselves in decision making can lead to caregiver burnout and even elder abuse. For example, if a care recipient needs 24-hour care, the caregiver may immediately think about how nice it would be for the loved one to stay at home as long as possible. What the caregiver does not think about is how this decision will impact him or her as the caregiver. Caregivers can find 24-hour care very demanding, especially if they have other responsibilities (i.e., spouse, adolescent children, work). Facing such demands, the caregiver may likely feel burned out and frustrated by the situation, and even lash out at the care recipient. The CFT therapist can help the caregiver think about all aspects of the options they generated while brainstorming ideas in order to make realistic assessments of the pros and cons of each option.

Caring for someone is a learning process. Some solutions may be successful, whereas others may not. It is important for therapists to reinforce a successful or effective outcome. The fourth step in rational problem solving is *evaluating outcomes of decisions and determining whether the best alternative was chosen.* When a caregiver implements a successful alternative, this leads to confidence in future problems-solving efforts (Nezu, Palmatier, & Nezu, 2004). On the other hand, if an outcome is less than optimal, it is important for the therapist to examine the process with the caregiver and discuss what may have impeded success.

In cases of cognitive impairment, CFT therapists sometimes coach their caregiver clients in a technique of *therapeutic lying,* which involves going along with the care recipient in their version of reality (see the example in Exhibit 3.2). For example, letting the care recipient believe that it is nighttime, even if it is morning (i.e., not arguing), can be soothing to the person with cognitive impairment. Alternatively, insisting that it is morning only heightens the person's confusion and disorientation, not to mention his or her agitation toward the caregiver. In the same sense, telling a person you are going for an ice cream cone and then going to a doctor's appointment may be a means of getting the older adult into the car without having to engage in a struggle, and once the person is at the physician's office, he or she will likely refrain from "making a scene" in the parking lot. Indeed, if this strategy is used only when the care recipient's cognitive impairment precludes all reasoning with them, the time lapse during the drive may have been sufficiently distracting that the person no longer is resistant to the doctor. If caregivers insist that their consciences will not allow them to "lie" to their care recipients, the CFT therapist can encourage them to follow through with the original promise. After the physician's appointment, the caregiver and care recipient can enjoy the ice cream cone.

An alternative frame is telling the care recipient's emotional truth, which sometimes requires the caregiver to select language that conveys truth to the care recipient differently than would be chosen for a person without cognitive impairment (Feil, 1993). For example, parents often tailor answers to the question, "Where do babies come from?" to be

EXHIBIT 3.2

Mary Ann

Mary Ann is a 30-year-old caregiver for her 85-year-old grandfather, James, who has been diagnosed with Alzheimer's disease. As his disease progressed and his functioning declined, Mary Ann moved in with her grandfather in order to provide 24-hour care. Recently, he had begun telling Mary Ann that he wanted to go home, that it was time to leave the barracks. Mary Ann found these situations to be very troubling because her grandfather was home, despite what he was reporting, but no amount of reasoning could convince him. Furthermore, this level of disorientation suggested additional decline in her loved one. He truly believed that he was in the army barracks and could describe them in great detail.

At first, she decided to reason with him and tell him that they were home and that he was just imagining the barracks, hoping that he would "snap out of it" once someone told him the truth. Her attempts at reasoning with him were met with frustration and anger because her grandfather was convinced that she was lying to him. Because of the disease progression, he simply lost the ability to reason critically. They would argue, and both Mary Ann and her grandfather would leave the arguments upset and emotionally exhausted.

After Mary Ann described her arguments with her grandfather to her CFT therapist, they engaged in a brainstorming activity. Mary Ann thought of calling her mother and having her grandfather speak with her on the phone (after coaching her mother to reassure her father that he was indeed living with Mary Ann). She also thought of having her grandfather look outside for cues about his environment. The therapist added that Mary Ann's grandfather might not be able to process the fact that he was not living in the barracks, and one solution might be for Mary Ann to "go along with" her grandfather's beliefs.

Mary Ann and her therapist generated a list of pros and cons associated with each of the ideas they had come up with related to her grandfather's belief that he was living in the barracks. The pros of calling her mother were that her grandfather was usually soothed by her mother's voice and that he enjoyed their conversations. The con was that her mother was generally asleep at the time when Mary Ann's grandfather was most agitated. One pro of having her grandfather look outside was that it was a convenient intervention, but the con was that using this strategy in the past had not had much impact on her grandfather's beliefs or his frustration level. A pro of going along with her grandfather's beliefs was the potential for less arguing and contention between them, and a con, Mary Ann felt, was that she would have to lie to her grandfather.

Reevaluating her initial less-than-optimal outcome, Mary Ann decided to try joining with him in what he was seeing—in his truth—the next time her grandfather asked to go home. She pretended that her twin bed in the other room was a car. She helped him into the "car" and when they "arrived home," she helped him out. Her grandfather was calm and even thanked her. Several hours later, her grandfather again asked to be taken home and Mary Ann successfully went through the same scenario again. No fighting, no problem.

Other possible solutions could have included actually driving her grandfather around the block or asking him to engage in certain activities to help distract him from his current dilemma of getting home. Having successfully handled the problem, Mary Ann will be likely to address the next problem with more confidence.

age appropriate for the child asking the question. A 6-year-old would be answered quite differently than a medical student studying reproductive science. We teach caregivers to respond to the underlying emotional question at the level of cognitive complexity that addresses the care recipient's concern. We encourage them to consider this telling the truth rather than lying because they are answering a care recipient's questions in ways that he or she can use. Thus, a caregiving spouse who tells her husband that they are headed out for a drive to see a nice man is communicating the safety and familiarity that is no longer communicated by telling him that they are going to see the "doctor." The skills of approaching problems from a positive orientation and implementing rational problem-solving strategies are generally taught by therapists through didactic explanations, skills training activities, role-play exercises, and homework assignments (Nezu, 2004).

Teaching a caregiver to implement the steps of the rational problem-solving approach eventually supports caregivers in becoming more and more positively oriented, especially as their self-efficacy increases and they learn that they can come up with effective solutions to problems (see the example in Exhibit 3.3). Further, the CFT therapist must also help caregivers to approach problems as challenges and not to avoid making decisions or working toward finding solutions to problems, and not to haphazardly or impulsively jump into decision making when problems arise. The more effective problem solvers caregivers become, the more confidence they will have in their caregiving abilities.

EXHIBIT 3.3

John

John was worried that his mother was becoming depressed because she so seldom left her house now that she had to carry oxygen and use a wheelchair. His mother had quit going to social engagements altogether, and she had begun asking him to do her grocery shopping unless she could run quickly into the store for an item or two at a time. After learning problem-solving techniques in caregiver family therapy, John decided to try the techniques with his mother. He asked his mother to help him generate solutions to getting her out of the house more often, frankly, because he was unsure why she wasn't engaging as she had previously. His mother said that she had difficulty carrying her oxygen tank even for short distances and that was why she would only take very short trips. Finally understanding his mother's difficulty, John was able to brainstorm with her ideas about how to troubleshoot so that she could participate more fully in her life.

John called the oxygen supplier and requested that two small oxygen tanks be delivered each week in addition to the current order. He and his mother also took a shopping trip together and picked out a pretty bag in which his mother could easily carry the smaller oxygen tanks. After problem solving together, John noticed that his mother seemed happier as she went back to her previous activities and routine.

To work through the problem-solving process, the CFT therapist asks the caregiver to think about a particular problem related to his or her caregiver role and to go through PST steps. The therapist should be helpful in generating possible solutions, particularly those solutions informed by a diagnosis or functional assessment. For example, a common solution for problem behaviors caused by dementia is distraction because the disease progression eliminates traditional reasoning skills that caregivers would have relied on previously in their relationship with the care recipient. Solutions that focus on reasoning are likely to be unsuccessful in persons with dementia, yet the caregiver who is a spouse or daughter will need a solution that is congruent with his or her desire to respect and protect the dignity of a loved one. Therapists usually need to role-play the use of distraction techniques in order for the family member to trust that distraction can be done effectively while honoring the familial roles of the caregiver and care recipient. After the role-play, discuss the thoughts that might become a barrier to using distraction. Respectful alternatives to "He should know what he is doing is wrong" and "I can't tell my father what to do" might be "Reasoning with him makes him more frustrated" and "He is so relieved when I can turn his attention away from the problem and we end up enjoying each other more than when he gets frustrated with my explanations."

After deciding on a course of action, ask the caregiver to try it at home and come back to discuss the results. Framing the next opportunity to try the chosen solution as an experiment frees the caregiver from feeling obligated to do it right the first time and keeps the door open to assisting him or her with tweaking implementation strategies. Furthermore, many strategies work only in particular contexts, and the first failure should lead to questions about the context rather than a wholesale rejection of the solution as viable. If the solution worked, it is important to discuss the success and the caregiver's willingness to do it again if a situation calls for it. If the solution did not work, explore the possible causes and review where skills could be improved.

PROBLEMS IMPLEMENTING PST IN FAMILIES

When making changes in care structures for the care recipient, a caregiver must think through several considerations. One is the care recipient's reactions to those changes. Another factor is the availability of family and community resources to offset some of the responsibilities of the primary caregiver; related to this are the demands placed on the caregiver and other family members to meet the needs of the care recipient. If only one member of the family lives in close proximity to the care recipient, and no other care supports are available, then much of the caregiving responsibilities will fall to the nearby caregiver. At the same time, if that caregiver is involved in multiple roles—wife, parent to children living at home, employee—this will limit the amount of time and energy the caregiver has to provide support to the care recipient. In such a situation, the CFT therapist may explore alternative arrangements with the caregiver, such as having the care recipient relocated to live near other available caregivers for some portion of time, looking into community living environments that provide some level of support or oversight for older adults, and/or having the caregiver look at their other roles and responsibilities to determine which, if any, might be reduced during the most intensive periods of caregiving.

Caregivers struggle at times to find the optimal level of involvement in the lives of their care recipients, even as they recognize that practical problems must be solved and, more than likely, solved by someone in the family. CFT therapists can help caregivers determine whether the help they offer is enough or whether their care recipient needs increased supports. Some caregivers may find themselves offering more help than necessary, which can be detrimental to both the caregiver and care recipient.

Day-to-day challenges encountered by care recipients can be signs that the caregiver needs to increase supports for the care recipient. For example, if a care recipient lives alone, and the caregiver finds that the number of phone calls he or she is receiving is increasing daily—to the point that the caregiver's other responsibilities are being interrupted—this is a sign that increased interaction with the care recipient is becoming necessary. If a caregiver repeatedly visits the care recipient and finds his or her refrigerator empty of nutritious food, then the caregiver can deduce that more support with shopping (and perhaps with cooking) are becoming necessary. Furthermore, if a care recipient repeatedly gets sick with the same symptoms or illness, the caregiver may begin to suspect that the care recipient needs increased support with managing physician appointments and/or medication administration. An accumulation of such examples suggests that increased supports and care may be needed, whether those will ultimately be supplied by the caregiver or through formal or informal care structures.

On the other end of the spectrum, consider a daughter whose mother lives with her and for whom the daughter cooks, cleans, arranges all appointments, and drives. In some situations, this high level of care may be necessary, such as toward the end of the caregiving journey, when the care recipient is significantly impaired and is truly unable to care for herself in any but the most rudimentary of capacities. However, if the mother in this situation simply preferred having her daughter "take care" of her and was reluctant to engage in activities that she was clearly still capable of accomplishing, then the therapist would likely want to encourage the caregiver to allow her mother to do more for herself.

Engaging in self-care, as well as other activities, helps to stimulate care recipients and keep them healthier longer (Tighe et al., 2008). Finding the best balance of involvement, one that keeps the care recipient safe and active, while allowing the caregiver time to fulfill other roles and responsibilities, is essential to the family as a whole.

In some cases, what seems to be an optimal solution for the caregiver and care recipient may turn out to cause problems for the larger family system. A mother of two teenage daughters may increase the time she spends taking her mother to appointments but over time may realize that her daughters are relying more and more on friends for rides to their activities. In general, the mother may not see this as a problem, but after a few months she may notice some strain between her and her daughters and may realize suddenly that the time she had previously spent driving them around town was one of the primary chances she had to capture their attention and spend quality time talking with them about how things were going in their lives. Role structuring to meet the care recipient's and the family's needs is discussed in more detail in Chapters 4 and 7.

Referring the Caregiver to Other Resources

Therapists need to be prepared to provide referrals to resources for solving problems outside the therapist's scope of knowledge and expertise. When a therapist is new to a community or unfamiliar with the practice of this type of therapeutic intervention, community resources, such as social workers or professional geriatric care managers, can be recommended to assist families in practical aspects of care for their loved one. A national resource is http://www.eldercare.gov, which helps families find the local Area Agency on Aging (AAA). Visitors to this website are prompted to put in the zip code for the older adult's home and are given contact information for the nearest AAA, where they can get information about resources in their area. One caveat that must be noted is that people will typically get what they ask for when calling AAAs. If they want a list of assisted living facilities, that is easy. If they want to know how to help a parent, then they need more than a list, so the caregiver will probably need to find a geriatric care manager to help figure it out.

A critical element for any professional working with caregivers in aging families is the need to respect the profound nature of the challenges that these families face when trying to obtain practical information to guide their decision making. Though one might presume that such resources would be readily available from health care professionals, they rarely provide such information.

CFT therapists also need to know about assistive technology resources, an emerging area of research and intervention strategies for individuals living with chronic disease. In an effort to support the independence of persons with chronic problems, we need to know about the technologies that can support development. A resource that helps identify and locate funding resources for assistive technology is the Assistive Technology Partners website (http://www.ucdenver.edu/academics/colleges/medicalschool/programs/atp/Pages/Assistive TechnologyPartners.aspx). CFT therapists can research online for assistive technology resources in their geographical locations as well.

Who Gets to Decide What Options to Consider for Structuring Care?

The CFT therapist and caregiver can work together to create a list of areas in which the care recipient needs additional support or structure to maintain an optimal level of functioning and use the rational problem-solving methods described previously to implement new strategies for care recipients to complete instrumental activities of daily living (IADLs) and activities of daily living (ADLs), maintain social activities, and remain safe in their environments at home and in the community. When the care recipient can participate meaningfully in these conversations, the caregiver should engage him or her in identifying preferences about how care will be structured. Even in early stages of dementia, care recipients are often still able to make choices and demonstrate their preferences. Later, simpler preference statements can still be made in response to simplified cues (LeBlanc, Cherup, Feliciano, & Sidener, 2006). Only when the person cannot participate in choosing safely does an advanced directive give authority to someone else to choose for the person. Specific legal criteria are established for invoking advanced directives, which must be determined by an appropriate health professional according to procedures and criteria established in state law. A more detailed discussion of how this process works in families is found in Chapter 9.

In families with multiple members involved in caregiving, many people may want input into care structures and decisions. The CFT client needs to be asked who is already involved, and who should be included in the decisions. Processes for engaging families in working together to structure care roles are discussed in detail in Chapter 4.

Addressing Specific Concerns

At this point, the focus of CFT is on identifying the care recipient's care needs and potential strategies for meeting them. Once these needs are identified, the process of structuring care roles can begin.

SOCIAL NEEDS OF THE CARE RECIPIENT

Social needs of older adults vary such that some individuals prefer talking with or visiting others throughout much of the day, every day, and others are satisfied with a few phone calls per week. Families have a historical relationship with the care recipient against which they compare the current social activity pattern and may become concerned if current behavior looks different from the past. Reduced social contact may be a natural or secondary consequence of a frail person's adaptation to mobility problems or limited physical energy. Sensory impairments, such as hearing and vision loss, may also impact an older adult's ability to engage socially. On the other hand, social withdrawal may reflect the fact that when a person is depressed, he or she may not necessarily desire increased social interaction. Unfortunately, social withdrawal also tends to perpetuate depression.

Families may not recognize that another cause of social withdrawal is cognitive impairment, which reduces a person's ability to initiate even desirable activities. Such failure to initiate interaction in social situations reduces opportunities to interact and makes the person appear withdrawn in social situations or uninterested in group activities. However, when positioned for a low-stimulation social context, the person may engage with obvious enjoyment of activities and interaction with others. Therefore, family members need to go back to the name of the problem to understand the cause of social withdrawal and to respond accordingly by problem solving the barriers to successful social interaction.

The caregiver can begin by asking, "What would this person enjoy?" and "What stands in the way of him or her doing it?" Holiday gatherings can be a miserable place for a person with cognitive impairment, depression, or hearing loss, but a wonderful place for a person with mobility problems who withdraws socially because of physical accessibility issues. A person with cognitive impairment needs a less stimulating place to be during the gathering (not at the center of the table). A person with hearing loss needs to be in a quiet corner, where people can come by one by one or a few at a time to chat. A depressed person needs to be allowed to engage but not pushed using a cheerleading style to appear happy. Knowing exactly why a person struggles in social situations can lead to appropriate problem solving to meet that person's needs.

DECISION-MAKING CAPACITY

Families usually notice problems with decision-making capacity when a care recipient demonstrates poor judgment about health care, medication or financial management, or continued driving after repeated tickets or accidents. At such a time, a full neuropsychological assessment is useful and necessary to make an accurate determination about an older adult's capacity to make decisions on his or her own behalf (see Chapter 2).

Once it is determined that a care recipient is incapacitated, several options exist for ensuring that he or she has the necessary supports in place. Depending on the level of incapacity, the older adult may be determined capable of selecting a proxy decision maker but not of making other specific decisions. When capacity becomes compromised, caregivers almost always wish they had talked earlier about the care recipient's preferences related to their late-life and end-of-life care. At the time when the care recipient is already experiencing difficulties with memory, executive functioning, and other cognitive skills, it may be too late to engage him or her in these types of conversations in a meaningful way.

Once a care recipient is determined to lack capacity, advanced directives may be invoked on the basis of determination of incapacity in particular decision-making domains (e.g., medical or financial decision-making). In some cases, a full court-appointed guardianship may become necessary, especially if the care recipient is very insistent about making his or her own decisions despite obvious poor judgment that leaves him or her open to danger to self or others. More commonly, families navigate the transition to a legally recognized proxy decision maker taking responsibility for the basic safety and well-being of the care recipient. Having a family member or caregiver fulfill this role is usually preferable to engaging a court-appointed guardian, although highly conflicted or overwhelmed families may benefit from the role being assigned to an outside, objective party.

To gain knowledge and skill in this area, CFT therapists can access resources such as the National Association of Elder Law Attorneys; the Probate Section of their local Bar Associations; and American Psychological Association (APA) and American Bar Association (ABA) books for judges, attorneys, and psychologists. Family therapists comfortable working in this legal arena may want to explore career opportunities associated with probate court. Elder law is an integrated team setting that is not often recognized by family intervention professionals but has an important role to play in assessment and family interventions. Whether family therapists recognize it, they are involved in a virtual team in any case involving families who question one member's ability to make decisions appropriately. Additional information about the pragmatics of this work is contained in Chapter 9.

FINANCIAL MANAGEMENT

Unpaid bills, utility disconnect notices, and disorganized check registers are some of the initial signs of poor financial management. Of course, having access to a care recipient's mail and checkbook assumes that the care recipient would readily share financial information with his or her family member. For a person who has always managed his own financial accounts and has never shared information about personal assets, having someone else take over that responsibility may seem incredibly intrusive.

Marson and colleagues (Hebert & Marson, 2007) have demonstrated that financial management can be viewed on a continuum from simple to complex. CFT therapists need to be familiar with the continuum in order to ask useful questions about what a person can still do even if some skills are beyond them. A deteriorating condition such as dementia does not have a simple relationship to financial capacity. This is a highly technical area in which rights need to be protected, balanced by protection of safety. Families need help figuring out what a person can actually do today; in other words, financial capacity is not all or nothing. Marson's concepts can be useful to clinicians in conjunction with a careful evaluation of the care recipient's capabilities before anyone decides to restrict capacity. APA and ABA books on financial management can also help guide CFT therapists in this area of work (American Bar Association Commission on Law and Aging and American Psychological Association, 2005; 2006; 2008).

An initial step into making a transition in financial decision making may involve engaging care recipients in a discussion about whom they would want to help them in the event that they were no longer able to manage their own finances. When the family knows in advance that the care recipient prefers a legal or financial representative over involving a family member, then the caregiver can help to make those arrangements. A caregiver and care recipient can discuss when the caregiver would know that the care recipient needs help with paying bills and managing a bank account in advance of any problems arising so that the caregiver could step in and involve the financial assistant at the appropriate time. Regardless of who takes over financial responsibility for the care recipient, someone must step in in the event that services are being discontinued or the bank is calling about overdrafts.

Older adults can make legal arrangements to have particular people or entities designated as Financial Powers of Attorney. States vary in the term used for these roles, so state-specific knowledge is needed as to what is meant by guardian or conservator, for example. Documents must be drawn up and finalized at a time when the adult still has capacity to make these particular decisions. When the incapacitated person has not named someone, the courts usually appoint a guardian, presumably someone who knows the care recipient and might have a good idea about what his or her preferences would have been. Nonetheless, a person appointed by the courts may or may not be the person that the care recipient would have chosen on his or her own, if given the opportunity. Therefore, when a care recipient receives a diagnosis of cognitive impairment, CFT therapists encourage caregivers to have conversations with their care recipients about their preferences as early as is possible in the course of the cognitive decline, allowing care recipients to have as much control as possible in the choices made regarding their lives.

CFT therapists do not have to become legal experts or even neuropsychological evaluators of capacity. But they do need to learn how this process works in both the legal system and the health care system. Family members with concerns about capacity need help putting together a team of professionals who can help them navigate the legal process. Over time, the CFT therapist needs to build understanding of those processes in order to help families make sense of their experience. For example, the legal standards for cognitive capacity vary by the decision being made, so an older adult may be determined to lack capacity to manage her own finances but be judged with capacity to select the person who will manage them. This highly technical legal domain requires careful assessment by someone familiar with capacity standards as well as approaches to assessment of capacity. Families are unlikely to understand how and why this works and how to apply the information to their particular situation. With this knowledge, CFT therapists can be valuable members of the team.

RISK OF EXPLOITATION

Many older adults, and perhaps especially those who are cognitively impaired, are at risk of exploitation both by people they know and by strangers. In some of the most notorious cases (e.g., Brooke Astor and Mickey Rooney), close family members have taken assets from older adults, preying on their poor judgment, memory, and inability to make informed decisions. The care recipients in such cases typically have some type of cognitive impairment and are unaware of what is

Samuel

Samuel was worried about his mother, Darla, who lived in a neighborhood filled with young families and single young men and in which most of the houses were rentals. He decided he would go by her house after work every day to check in on her and sort through her mail with her to decide what correspondence was important and what could be discarded. He asked his mother every day whether she had had any visitors because he realized that when he waited 2 or 3 days to ask, Darla always said that she could not remember whether anyone had been by to see her.

occurring (Wilber & Reynolds, 1997). In other situations, sweepstakes, television commercials, phone solicitors, and people in the community are involved in the exploitation of older adults by selling items or services that the older adult does not need or that are never delivered.

Even among persons with intact cognition, other factors enhance risk of exploitation and mistreatment. Older adults with physical vulnerabilities may rely on family members for practical help and fear the consequences of losing that assistance if they confront inappropriate actions (Hafemeister, 2003). Other family members simply feel responsible for the exploitive person who is himself or herself impaired. A common profile of an exploitive family member is someone who is actually dependent on the older adult because of physical or psychological difficulties (P. Jones, 1996; O'Neill & Flanagan, 1998). Other characteristics include presence of psychopathology, alcohol or substance abuse, and unemployment (Dessin, 2000; Tueth, 2000). Complex family dynamics are at work in such situations in which older adults feel protective of the very people exploiting them (C. M. Beck & Ferguson, 1981).

At particular risk are older family members who live alone. People who live in communities with other older adults and assisted living facilities may have some built-in supports for protection. A person seeking to take advantage of older adults may be more likely to target those who are isolated, have fewer visitors, and have less oversight (Choi & Mayer, 2000; Nerenberg, 2008). Accordingly, additional steps may be needed to protect older family members who live alone (see the example in Exhibit 3.4).

HEALTH CARE MANAGEMENT

Poor health care management can result in physical illness or decline in functioning. In some cases, caregivers will need to obtain Medical Powers of Attorney to become decision makers for a care recipient who truly lacks capacity. As with other ADLs and IADLs, a full assessment of a person's functioning level is needed before assuming that a person

EXHIBIT 3.5

Melissa

Melissa understood that poor hygiene is a common problem with persons with dementia, but she was not sure what to do about it. Melissa's father had been reluctant to shower for the past few weeks, and he had stopped shaving altogether. Melissa's CFT therapist expanded on some of the findings of her father's recent neuropsychological assessment, explaining that deficits in executive functioning often translated into poor initiation of daily activities. Once Melissa understood why her father's routine was disrupted, she arranged a system of prompts, including signs on the bathroom door saying "shower in the morning" along with a picture of the bathtub for her father.

is incapable of making medical decisions on his or her own behalf (see the example in Exhibit 3.5). Before seeking Medical Power of Attorney, caregivers can try problem-solving methods to approach a care recipient's poor health care management. For example, a person with diabetes typically sees a physician three to four times a year, depending on how well he or she manages the diabetes symptoms. Other medical illnesses also require monitoring and oversight by a physician, so an inability to call a physician's office, make an appointment, and follow through with going to that appointment is a sign that more support is needed in this domain of functioning, especially for older adults with chronic health concerns.

We all know people who hate going to the doctor and will almost always refuse a trip to the physician unless they are in serious pain or are fearful about their symptoms. In these cases, encouragement to attend a yearly physical and offering to drive the care recipient to the appointment may be all that is needed in terms of caregiver involvement. However, a visit to the physician is necessary and perhaps even urgent for individuals experiencing unusual symptoms, unexplained weight loss or gain, changes in sleep patterns, or any other type of physical change that is concerning. In such cases, even when a care recipient refuses medical care, the caregiver must not wait for the care recipient's compliance to schedule and have them attend an appointment with their health care provider.

CFT therapists at times have to coach caregivers through conversations with their care recipients by role-playing. When a care recipient is adamant about not going to see his or her physician, and when the care recipient is at serious medical risk, the caregiver may have few choices about how to handle the situation. Options include offering to take the care recipient to his or her favorite activity after the doctor's appointment and/or calling the physician and having him or her tell the care recipient over the phone to come in for a visit. Further intervention may be necessary, which at first glance may feel extreme or too difficult: telling the care recipient you are taking him or her somewhere other than the physician's office and then taking him or her to the doctor anyway or calling emergency responders when the physical risk to the care recipient is high. Therapists need to help family caregivers choose the least intrusive approach possible and to identify strategies for implementing it that are respectful. Role-playing is an ideal way of modeling respect through tone, body language, and words. Many times, caregivers literally cannot picture interacting with their family member in totally new ways, so therapists need to provide multiple models from which the caregiver can choose an option.

MEDICATION ADMINISTRATION

Inconsistent medication administration may show up as recurring medical illness or rapid change in symptoms or functional abilities. Medication mismanagement can easily produce a delirium state that may appear to families primarily as confusion, frequent falling, excessive sleepiness, or agitation. Poorly managed symptoms may be more a problem of inappropriate medication administration than a poor treatment plan.

As with all other practical problems, the first step is to identify the underlying cause of the problem. Medication mismanagement can occur because a person has a lifelong paranoia about the medical-pharmaceutical industry that leads him or her to resist taking any medication regularly, or it may be due to something as simple as trouble swallowing. Alternatively, a person with memory problems may have trouble remembering whether morning medications were taken and deal with that uncertainty by retaking them or not taking them "just in case." Some older adults notice side effects that frighten or concern them and lead them to change their medication regimen without telling anyone. Still others self-medicate with alcohol or over-the-counter medications that produce problematic side effects or undermine the efficacy of the prescription medication. The list of potential problems with medication administration is almost endless, so a careful assessment of the exact medication administration pattern (what is taken when, with what food/drink) is a key piece of information that needs to be combined with the background information gathered in the naming step of CFT to form a reasonable hypothesis about the cause of the specific mismanagement problem.

A fairly unobtrusive method of managing medication self-administration is to assist the care recipient with filling a "medication reminder" box with their daily pills. These boxes can be as simple as seven small connected containers, one for each day of the week, or 28 containers that allow for morning, noon, afternoon, and evening medications each day for 7 days. Rather than waiting 1 month for the care recipient's prescription to run out, the caregiver can look each day to see whether medications have been taken as prescribed.

For older adults who do not have someone who can monitor medication self-administration, and for those who have already demonstrated that they are unable to manage this task, automated medication dispensing machines can dispense the appropriate medication at the scheduled time of day and sound an alarm for the older adult to take his or her medications. These boxes can be helpful, but they may be somewhat costly. Agencies also exist that will send a home-care nurse to the house of the care recipient for the express purpose of monitoring medication administration.

Medication administration problems that occur because of a deliberate decision on the part of the older adult need to be handled differently. The prescriber needs to negotiate the treatment plan to identify an approach to disease and symptom management that is acceptable to the patient. Family members may need to offer support and advocacy to assist with this process, ensuring that the older adult has been heard and taken seriously regarding preferences. An ideal medication may need to be switched for a less effective one if the latter offers a more tolerable set of side effects. Families may help the older adult communicate preferences, practices (e.g., over-the-counter medications, vitamins), or difficulties (e.g., swallowing, incontinence that leads to underhydration) that the health care provider simply could not otherwise know.

NUTRITION AND COOKING

To determine whether increased supports are needed with nutrition and cooking, a caregiver will want to observe food intake patterns and monitor access to nutrition. Families sometimes simply need to look in the refrigerator and cupboards. Expired and moldy foods are indicators that an older adult is not monitoring what he or she has on hand, and eating these items could cause serious illness. If the care recipient does not have any fresh foods on hand, that may also be a sign that he or she has not been to the store recently. A freezer full of frozen dinners and ice cream is probably not sufficient to meet the nutritional needs of anyone. One consideration, however, is that if the person has always lived on frozen dinners, a lack of food in the refrigerator may not be a cause for concern. A caregiver might notice that his or her family member has shifted to eating only soft foods because of difficulty chewing, at which point an appointment with a dentist could help address any problems with dentition. Another factor to consider is access to transportation. A person may have a lack of fresh foods simply because he or she does not have a way of getting to the store, as opposed to being unable to plan and execute a shopping trip. Another indicator of difficulties with nutrition and cooking is burned or discarded food or cooking utensils and pans.

A person may begin having difficulty with cooking because of memory or executive functioning impairments, which can lead to a person walking away from a pot on the stove and not remembering he or she was cooking. Ultimately, weight loss, dehydration, and other physical illnesses may be signals of malnutrition associated with difficulties with maintaining nutritious eating and cooking.

Older adults may have difficulty with cooking for other reasons, so the underlying cause of the difficulty needs to be understood before problem solving is attempted. Persons who lack ability to stand long enough to prepare foods could benefit from instruction in cooking quick and easy meals. For people who have difficulty cooking with a stove and oven because of memory problems, one intervention that may prove helpful is leaving instructions for cooking favorite meals in the microwave. Those with vision impairments may need large type labels on easy-to-open containers maintained in exact locations. Cooking with another family member is probably the safest intervention of all (see the example in Exhibit 3.6).

Finally, some people simply cannot access the grocery store to buy food but could prepare meals if food arrived in the home. Family members may shop for the older adult in such cases or identify grocery stores with delivery services. Senior services agencies assist older adults in getting to stores through their transportation programs and by bringing food to their homes through programs such as Meals on Wheels. Some of these agencies charge low fees for their services, and some are funded by grants and donations and are therefore free to people who qualify. When the care recipient is able to successfully heat meals in the microwave, the caregiver still needs to monitor nutrition and cooking abilities in some cases in order to make sure that when the microwave

---

EXHIBIT 3.6

Paul

After being diagnosed as prediabetic, Paul lost interest in food altogether. He stopped shopping and cooking for himself, skills he had been managing well since becoming a widower several years earlier. His son noticed the change and arranged for him and Paul to attend nutrition and cooking classes together at a local health promotion clinic. Soon, Paul was back to himself, and even though he said he did not enjoy food as much as he had in the past, he acknowledged that sharing mealtimes with his son a few times a week was encouraging and pleasant to him.

---

becomes too difficult for the care recipient to operate, new strategies for healthy eating can be implemented.

FALLS AND PHYSICAL SAFETY

Bruises and bumps, broken bones, and head injuries are all consequences of falls. Vision impairment, in particular, puts older adults at an exceptional risk of falling. Older adults often struggle with balance and mobility, and many try to continue activities they "could always do" far beyond their ability to engage in those behaviors safely. Imagine a person who recently had surgery now attempting to trim trees, stand on a ladder to paint or hang pictures, walk on wet or slippery surfaces, or even climb stairs. Some behaviors that probably seem safe enough but can pose extreme safety risks include showering without handrails and shower mats and using a stepstool to reach something on a high shelf.

Although it can be a difficult transition for some (see the example in Exhibit 3.7), requesting that older adults ask for help with household tasks rather than trying to do them on their own (especially when no one else is home) can go a long way toward preventing falls and other physical injuries. Having a notepad in an easily accessible place, where the care recipient can jot down a "to do" list for a caregiver or hired staff may be one helpful strategy for preventing falls. Making sure that the caregiver is accessible and willing to help with household chores (or able to hire someone to help with these tasks) is another important factor in inviting care recipients to wait for help. No one wants to rely on someone who always appears too busy to help. Hiring nearby children and teens to help with the upkeep of the yard and snow removal can be an excellent way both to keep the older adult from trying to complete these household maintenance tasks themselves and also engaging the care recipient in some interaction with younger people in the neighborhood.

The caregiver can be as creative as possible in finding less risky tasks for the older adult to engage in that are both meaningful and fulfilling while also supporting the role of overseer of the hired staff. Although

---

EXHIBIT 3.7

Betty

Betty was caring for her husband, who had a penchant for doing very dangerous household maintenance tasks, including climbing trees to trim branches, painting his house, and repairing his roof. Even in midstage dementia, with a history of frequent falls because of poor balance, he was constantly at risk of falling and sustaining serious injuries. Yet, he viewed Betty as a nag when she tried to talk him out of doing these tasks. He had always been in charge of household maintenance and was not about to give up that role.

---

lawn mowing may become too strenuous a task for some older adults, a person who always enjoyed yard work may still want to tend a garden during the summertime, especially if the caregiver joins in the activity with the care recipient and makes it a joint endeavor.

The therapist sometimes needs to help the caregiver assess carefully the level of risk to the care recipient. Some caregivers are overly protective and assess risk inaccurately or have such low tolerance that the care recipient may be discouraged from doing tasks that are healthy and appropriate. Once again, approaching the question of how much risk is appropriate requires a clear understanding of the problem and a solid problem-solving analysis of pros and cons of various solutions.

DRIVING

Driving is a very common safety concern for caregivers, families, and therapists, and at times for older adults themselves. The first question for the CFT therapist is whether there is clear evidence that driving is a risk. Family members may be wary and overly cautious, noting driving errors that are lifelong or insufficient to signal a need for change in driving privileges. The therapist needs to listen carefully for the evidence that there is a problem and link it to what is known about the care recipient's health conditions. Any problem the family observes should have a clear etiology that cannot be addressed to improve safety risks.

Once a clear picture has emerged that is founded on assessments of cognitive or physical capacity, the CFT therapist needs to help the family identify strategies for restricting driving. Only the rare care recipient willingly hangs up her car keys and decides driving is no longer within her skill set. Caregivers not only struggle with the idea of reducing the care recipient's independence by taking away the keys, but they also frequently meet a significant amount of resistance to the idea by the care recipient. Further, caregivers who are able to limit or cease driving by the impaired care recipient also have the responsibility of either providing or finding alternative transportation for the care recipient.

Who will evaluate driving skill specifically, and who will act to restrict driving privileges? Of course, some older adults become scared of their own driving and reluctant to get out on the road. Families may be able to persuade a person with awareness of their limitations to restrict the places or times that they drive. For example, a person with vision impairments that reduce nighttime acuity may choose not to drive at night. More challenging are persons who fail to recognize the risks of their impairments, such as intense fatigue, fluctuations in oxygen saturation or glucose levels, or dementia.

A driving evaluation is often a useful step in the process of imposing driving restrictions. Rules and regulations surrounding safe driving and driver's licenses vary from state to state, so it is essential that the CFT therapist is familiar with laws in their areas. In some states, the department of motor vehicles will reassess older adults' driving abilities on a more frequent basis after a certain age has been reached. If this is not the case in the area where you live, other options are still available to caregivers to assess an older adult's abilities to drive safely. Driving courses and assessments are offered in most urban areas, and if the caregiver and care recipient live far away from any of these companies, a trip to the nearest city for an evaluation may be warranted, given the risks of driving beyond one's capacity to do so. Physicians may also be willing to communicate with care recipients about their driving when caregivers are concerned. Furthermore, many rehabilitation programs within hospitals offer driving evaluations.

Families need to address the implications of driving restrictions on the person's everyday life. Making the decision to stop the care recipient from driving has different implications in rural areas than in cities, where public transportation is more readily available. Knowing whether the immediate area has transportation services, such as city buses or transit systems or services specifically tailored for older adults, is essential in making decisions about changing care structures around driving. Busses, city-run transportation systems, and taxis are other alternatives. Some transportation agencies are specifically tailored for older adults and will pick them up at their homes and take them to appointments and other activities. Some senior centers, senior service agencies, and Programs of All-Inclusive Care of the Elderly may also provide transportation to and from their site-based activities and physicians' appointments. In rural areas, transportation may not be as readily available, but creative problem solving may help increase alternatives, such as having neighbors take the care recipient shopping when they are going, asking friends from church to stop by on their way and taking the care recipient to church with them, and having the caregiver stop by more frequently.

ELDER ABUSE

Like exploitation, elder abuse occurs between care recipients and people they know as well as people they do not know. Cooper, Blanchard, Selwood, Walker, and Livingston (2010) found that one third of caregivers who were referred for psychiatric care reported they had significantly abused their care recipients, and half of the caregivers reported they had engaged in some abuse. Physical injuries, poor hygiene, unexplained weight loss, and emotional problems are some of the signs that the care being provided is not adequate or, in some cases, that abuse may be occurring. Although these caregivers are a select subsample of all caregivers, the rate of abuse is alarming. Recent prevalence rates have suggested that elder abuse and neglect affects an estimated 4.6% of individuals over the age of 65 (Acierno et al., 2010).

When caregivers first come in for therapy, they sign an Informed Consent and Mandatory Disclosure document that states the conditions under which a client's privilege of confidentiality is waived. Therapists must ensure that the client understands that the therapist must report situations in which the caregiver discloses that he or she is a danger to self or others, when abuse has occurred, or when the client becomes so gravely impaired that he or she is a risk to self or others. When a CFT therapist suspects that a client or a care recipient is in danger of abuse or neglect, the therapist must call the police and/or the Department of Human Services' Adult Protective Services in that region to ensure the safety of the parties involved. When the CFT therapist calls the local authorities, this could disrupt the therapeutic relationship to such a degree that the caregiver may not want to continue in therapy. Therefore, it is wise for the CFT therapist to tell the client that they must call the police and/or Adult Protective Services, to make sure that the caregiver understands the therapist's legal obligation to protect the care recipient, and to offer the caregiver an opportunity to make the call on his or her own (from the therapist's office so that the therapist knows that the call has been completed). Regardless of the client's reaction, the CFT therapist is obligated to make the call. The pragmatics of abuse reporting are discussed also in Chapter 9.

DISCUSS FUTURE PLANNING

Systematic planning can increase problem-solving effectiveness. Developing a plan reduces uncertainty by specifying who will do what under what circumstances. Planning can also lead to better problem resolution, which ultimately leads to less distress and better overall coping (Houts et al., 1996). One planning aspect that should be covered with all caregivers is what will happen to the care recipient if something happens to the caregiver. Often, caregivers are so focused on being ready to handle any problem that comes up today that they forget to consider what would happen to their loved one if they could not be there (i.e., in the case of an emergency or an accident). The therapist will want to encourage the caregiver to talk to other family members or trusted friends and make those plans. We often tell caregivers that it is great to hope for the best in life, but we should be prepared for the worst.

DISCUSS THE UNKNOWNS

The therapist and caregiver will find it impossible to address every possible aspect of and detail about the caregiving situation. We cannot fully know what will happen tomorrow for any of us, so acknowledging this with the caregiver and then planning for unknowns is one of the most important interventions in CFT. Gentle but complete explorations of reasonably likely *what if*s (what could happen, what might happen, and worst-case scenarios) during therapy sessions can help caregivers prepare for the inevitable bumps in the road they will encounter during their caregiving journeys.

Quick Tips for Addressing ADLs and IADLs

Caregivers may need to increase supports for their care recipients in many different areas of functioning, often referred to as ADLs. Many of these are examined below, with a focus on implementing the problem-solving process in the development of alternative care structures. The suggestions that follow are just one set of possibilities, and in general, caregivers are usually very good at developing and testing alternative solutions to difficult situations, particularly when they are approaching problems from a positive orientation. CFT therapists encourage and teach caregiver clients to develop a positive orientation by noticing caregivers' strengths (and pointing them out), by providing empathy, and also by challenging caregivers' negative self-statements and emotions that tend to hinder problem-solving efforts. Judicious references to other caregivers who have solved problems can provide a peer model that may offer hope that practical problems can be addressed successfully by real people in real situations, not just by professionals, yet avoid suggesting that everyone else solves problems easily.

The two commonly accepted categories of domains of everyday function that are used in senior care, health care, and rehabilitation services were introduced in Chapter 1 as markers of caregiving stages: activities of daily living and instrumental activities of daily living. These categories need to be understood by family caregivers for two reasons. Professionals use them in their acronym form (ADLs and IADLs) quite freely, so families benefit from knowing exactly what they mean. Equally important, families will find the list of ADLs and IADLs a useful reference point in their own efforts to oversee care. A more detailed description follows because these are the categories of care recipient needs around which most problem-solving work will be focused.

- IADLs are those skills needed to manage and structure independent lives. Examples include transportation, shopping, laundry, medication administration, food preparation, heavy household chores, making phone calls and appointments, financial management, and accessing community resources. IADLs require cognitive skills (e.g., planning, memory, initiation), social skills, and physical abilities to complete the tasks. Therefore, individuals who have cognitive impairment often begin to struggle with these types of abilities as their cognitive disorders progress. People with health problems and/or mental health concerns, such as depression, may also struggle with IADLs in that they may lack the physical strength or stamina needed, or they may lack the initiative to begin and complete them.

- ADLs are less complicated tasks than IADLs but require some level of physical strength and bodily control. The typical list of ADLs includes ambulation, transferring from one place to another (e.g., bed to chair), toileting, eating, bathing, and dressing and grooming.

To be safe, a person must be able to complete ADLs and IADLs independently or have adequate assistance from someone else. Much of the caregiving journey involves making sure that the care recipient's needs in these areas are sufficiently met and that supports increase at a consistent rate with the care recipient's decline in functioning.

Whether a care recipient has physical or cognitive impairments impacts the types of problems caregivers encounter. For example, in cases of cognitive impairment, dealing with the difficult behaviors of the loved one they are caring for is one of the biggest struggles caregivers face. Dressing, eating, bathing—basic activities of living—often become difficult to manage for both the care recipient and the caregiver. The caregiver may come to therapy specifically to figure out how to handle problem behaviors that arose during care tasks. Common examples include a mother who refuses to change clothes or a husband who hits his wife caregiver during bathing. In cases of physical impairment, caregivers may encounter practical challenges in providing care in the face of physical disability (e.g., bathing a person who cannot maintain upright posture). Difficult situations outside of these basic activities also can be stressful, such as a care recipient's stubborn refusal to make an appointment with the doctor that appears rooted in a lifelong personality pattern. CFT therapists should have concrete tips to provide a caregiver so that he or she can more effectively handle these inevitable situations. With this in mind, the therapist might often find it helpful to consider himself or herself as more of a coach than a therapist.

Here are some tips for caregivers of people with physical limitations:

- Bathing
  - Install grab bars next to toilets, bathtubs, and showers to prevent falls.

- Get a stool for the tub or shower or, at least, put a sturdy lawn chair right in the tub on a nonslip rubber mat.
- Get a hand-held shower attachment to make rinsing off possible while seated.
- Nutrition
  - Encourage foods that are high in calories and protein.
  - Offer small frequent snacks or meals (every couple of hours) on small plates to make the food appear less overwhelming.
  - Offer nutrient-dense foods like cheese and crackers, nuts, cottage cheese, and yogurt for snacks rather than focusing nutrition intake within three meals.
  - Use energy drinks, such as Ensure, to add nutritional value and to help people who may struggle with swallowing thinner liquids.
  - Encourage frequent hydration by making attractive liquids available constantly.
- Sleep problems
  - Encourage exercise during the day and limit daytime napping.
  - Set a quiet, peaceful tone in the evening to encourage sleep.
  - Restrict access to caffeine late in the day.

Here are some tips for caregivers of people with cognitive impairment:

- Bathing
  - Tell the person what you are doing prior to each step of the bath.
  - Substitute sponge baths for showers when feasible.
  - Coach the person through the steps of bathing to increase their sense of control of the situation.
  - Bathe the person as quickly and efficiently as possible while maintaining a soothing voice in a quiet, calm spa-like space.
- Dressing
  - Allow the person to choose from a limited selection of outfits. If he or she has a favorite outfit, consider buying several identical sets.
  - Arrange the clothes in the order in which they are to be put on to help the person move through the process.
  - Encourage the person to dress himself or herself to whatever degree possible using verbal or visual cues at each step. Plan to allow extra time, so there is no pressure or rush.
- Sleep problems
  - Try to keep bedtime at a similar time each evening. Routines, in general, can be very helpful to help structure the day for care recipients.
  - Ensure that the environment is safe in cases of nighttime wakefulness and wandering.

- ■ Visiting the doctor
  - ■ Schedule the appointment for the person's best time of day.
  - ■ Ask the office staff what time of day the office is least crowded to reduce likelihood of overstimulation.
  - ■ If rumination about pending appointments is a challenge, don't tell the person about the appointment until the day of the visit and even shortly before it is time to go.
  - ■ Be positive and matter-of-fact in stating that it is now time to go.
  - ■ Bring along a change of clothes in the event that clothing becomes soiled.
  - ■ Use distraction in the event that the care recipient becomes agitated, keeping distraction items available at all times.

This brief list of tips comes from a variety of sources, and although they have been separated by the types of difficulties the care recipient may have, many tips can overlap and be equally effective for people in varied situations. Many useful tips can also be found on the National Alliance for Caregiving (http://www.caregiving.org) and National Family Caregivers Association (http://www.nfcacares.org) websites, and others have come from organizations such as the National Institute on Aging (http://www.nia.nih.gov/) and the Alzheimer's Association (http://www.alz.org). Books on caregiving, such as *The 36-Hour Day* (Mace & Rabins, 2006) and *The Eldercare Handbook* (Henry & Convery, 2006), also contain helpful tips.

Conclusion

Given that older adults who are care recipients need care and support structures to be tailored for their individual needs, the CFT therapist assists families with transitioning into appropriate care models. CFT guides the caregiver in identifying care and support structures that are needed, drawing on information gathered during the naming process regarding diagnoses and functioning as well as family beliefs about the care recipient's problems. CFT therapists teach caregivers to solve problems from a positive orientation and practice rational problem-solving techniques to address a number of situations regarding the safety and well-being of care recipients. Good problem solving is the foundation for family role structuring activities that allocate the work of caregiving and to support good self-care by the caregivers.

Role Structuring | 4

F amilies often struggle with caregiving role transitions. Some family members find it challenging to take on the role of caregiver, whereas others find particular phases of caregiving challenging. Some family caregivers struggle to coordinate care with other family members, and others have trouble giving up the caregiving roles when it is time. And in most families, it is not a single caregiver who has to adjust—many members of a family may find themselves in new or different roles during the journey of caregiving to an elderly member.

Beyond the obvious workload of elder care, families struggle emotionally and interpersonally as members' aging evokes shifts in roles. Although not always recognized for the profound impact they have, caregiving roles engage families in new configurations of decision making, nurturance, and other core family dynamics. Clients who have been in individual psychotherapy for other reasons may bring challenges related to caregiving into the work. The caregiver family therapy (CFT) model can be applied usefully in that

DOI: 10.1037/13943-004
Caregiver Family Therapy: Empowering Families to Meet the Challenges of Aging,
by S. H. Qualls and A. A. Williams

individual psychotherapy context as well as in contexts in which service providers encounter families who explicitly seek services to help them make sense of the caregiving roles.

Within the sequence of tasks outlined in the CFT model, role transitions become the focus after the problem has been named and reasonably well understood, and the challenges of care begin to be addressed in practical ways. As described in Chapter 3 of this volume, caregivers are on a steep learning curve to address practical challenges, which have been compared with the demands of a new job (Aneshensel, Pearlin, Mullan, Zarit, & Whitlatch, 1995). Caregiving involves changes in roles that can range from minor tweaking of existing roles to very substantive changes in the structure or rules for one or more relationships. The intensity of the role change is determined by the needs of the care recipient: How much assistance does the caregiver need to provide or arrange for others to provide? Additionally, the well-being of the caregiver and the broader caregiving structure are also major factors. Alignment between the care recipient's needs and the caregiver's capability to meet those needs over time is key. The processes for identifying the amount of care needed have been detailed in previous chapters, so the focus here is on what to do once you recognize that a caregiver client needs to restructure roles in order to meet the care recipient's needs. As a reminder, Chapter 8 contains the cases that describe clinical work with Julio and Lupé as well as with Linda and Mrs. Johnson as illustrations of how this step in the therapy process can unfold.

Understanding the caregiving situation for which a particular person has sought help requires the therapist to have a broad frame for the family context of this caregiving moment. The pieces of that broader frame include the family structure, family development history, and caregiving role structures. Although many CFT therapists will work in settings that constrain the time available to gather such information, others will be able to pursue such information intentionally and may even gather it over longer periods of time. A psychologist working in primary care may gain insights into the family caregiver structure over a period of years, literally, at a rate of three or four appointments per year. A counselor in a social service agency may systematically gather family system information over a few weekly sessions, after which interventions elicit functional information as members of the family system respond to those interventions, thus demonstrating their system in action. Family interventions in care settings that limit therapy to very brief contacts require CFT therapists to apply even limited background information (e.g., number of children and ages of children living in the caregiving home, demands of job and other family roles) to hypothesize system issues that are likely to arise as the client's family addresses the needs of a frail family member.

In this chapter, we focus on the practical and emotional processes involved in accomplishing role transitions into, and through, caregiving situations in later life. We offer suggestions for assessing and intervening in family roles and role transitions, peppering our description with stories of caregivers with whom we have worked or cojourneyed.

Family Structures in Later Life

Later life families are typically very complex emotionally and organizationally, perhaps showing more complexity than at any other stage of the family life cycle. Certainly, they are drawing on the longest history of any family structure, a history of caring, struggling, competing, trying, wishing, pleading, supporting, stealing, giving, resenting, and so on. Longevity of family relationships provides more than enough time to create and resolve pain repeatedly over the course of a shared life span. Elder care, one of the most challenging normative transitions of later life, overlays all the existing complexity.

The structure of the family is the starting point for understanding options for caregiving. Who is in the family, in what relationships, with what changes over time in that structure? A clinical reality is that family structures are almost infinitely variable, with limitless possible combinations of marriages, partnerships, divorces, children born or adopted or fostered, deaths, cutoff relationships, and so on. Furthermore, sharing of residences or finances and collaborative business ventures can add complexity to structural relationships. Family therapists often use genograms to depict family structures because process challenges and opportunities can become visible in the mapping of the basic structures of a family (McGoldrick, Gerson, & Petry, 2008; see the example in Exhibit 4.1). Figure 4.1 shows an example genogram illustrating Exhibit 4.1.

Family structures include the actual legal relationships (marriages, divorces, births, deaths, adoptions) as well as the emotional relationship patterns of bonds, alliances, and conflicts. The CFT therapist needs to recognize the family membership and structure that is either unrelated to, or divergent from, the caregiving structure. Structural challenges that are readily visible on a genogram include complex partnership structures (e.g., marriages and remarriages, short-term cohabitation partnerships) and relationship cutoffs. Annotations to the genogram may also include boundary issues, such as enmeshments, overburdened individuals, and underbenefitted individuals. Resource issues, such as poverty or immigration and acculturation, may complicate caregiving. Also interesting are interracial or interethnic marriages or lesbian, gay,

---

EXHIBIT 4.1

Cathy

Cathy came to therapy with concern related to her mother's recent cognitive decline. Cathy's father died 1 year ago, and she had been checking in on her mother for the past 6 months after recognizing her deteriorating functioning. She stated that she has three sisters and one brother, all of whom lived in the area, but she was distraught and angry about their lack of involvement in caring for their mother. Cathy did not identify herself as her mother's "caregiver," but she knew that something had to be done in order to ensure her mother's safety. She stated that she was considering taking a leave of absence from her job in order to care for her mother full time, although she did not know if this was necessary or even her role to step in.

Cathy and her therapist drew a genogram in session to indicate all of the people in her mother's life, and then Cathy identified the nature of these relationships in the past (Figure 4.1). She described her brother as always being the outsider who never stepped up to the plate to help out. Her youngest sister was busy with her newly launched career and had told Cathy directly that she was simply too busy to help. However, Cathy had tried talking with her other two sisters about their mother's condition, but neither of them would commit either way. She also stated that her mother had one close friend, Margaret, who visited her mother every day and whom her mother trusted. Thus, Cathy drew lines between herself and her mother, and between her mother and Margaret, to indicate their close contact. She drew her brother and youngest sister as farther away from their mother because of their limited contact, and she drew dotted lines between her two other sisters and their mother, as she felt ambiguous about their roles. After drawing the family genogram, Cathy could easily see that her role was much more clearly defined than she had thought, and she was better able to identify herself as being a caregiver for her mother.

Note. From *The Aging Families and Caregiver Program: A Guide to Caregiver Family Therapy,* by L. Anderson, S. Horning, A. June, K. Kane, M. Marty, R. Pepin, and C. Vair, 2008, Unpublished manuscript. Copyright 2008 by L. Anderson, S. Horning, A. June, K. Kane, M. Marty, R. Pepin, and C. Vair. Reprinted with permission.

bisexual, or transgendered relationships that may challenge the family rules. Therapists need to be curious about how families have managed these structural challenges previously and how caregiving may further the challenge. In addition to structures, genograms can use symbols to depict process information about alliances, bonds, and conflicts, as well as historical information relevant to the family.

Geographic dispersion is an important factor in who provides what types of care within aging families, so it may be relevant to note on a genogram. We once interviewed a midlife daughter who lived with her family literally halfway around the world from her aging parents and her brother, whose behavior problems growing up were intrusive on her sense of safety and well-being. Her commitment to care for her aging parents was certainly influenced by geographic distance, but that geographic distance was also a clear (albeit not explicitly intentional) strategy to limit expectations of responsibilities for caregiving within the family.

Although all members may appear on a genogram as a set of circles and squares that look similar in size, all family members are not equal in potency for the caregiver client or care recipient. Individual differ-

FIGURE 4.1

Cathy

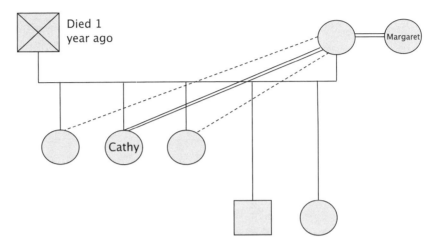

A genogram illustrating Exhibit 4.1.

ences of many types can be noted on a genogram, including health and mental health problems, personality traits, or any other characteristic that might seem relevant to the caregiving circumstance because of its potency to someone. The evolution of Linda's family genogram during the course of intervention illustrates the flexibility with which this tool can be used (see Chapter 8).

INTERVIEW TO ELICIT STRUCTURE INFORMATION

During the initial interview, the therapist asks about the current caregiving situation and asks for at least some family structure information as a backdrop to that caregiving information. Detailed information on family members and family structures needs to be noted to ensure that the information is not lost. Genograms are ideal ways to take notes because information fragments are immediately placed into relation to one another, and gaps in knowledge about family structure are readily apparent through missing structures. The therapist may show the caregiver client the partially constructed genogram, with a request to complete it or react to what is evident. Clients may shift perspective when they see the structures in black and white. Families are so familiar with their structures that they may not notice the aspects of family structure that are nonobvious (e.g., missing information about a person who is cut off from the family). For example, a simple question about the number of siblings in a family may elicit information about a previously unidentified family member whose absence is a source of great distress. Jotting down the city in which members reside can make it obvious to the therapist that members who are geographically available are surprisingly uninvolved or members who are far distant are significant decision makers despite having little information about day-to-day functioning. In other words, the process of developing the genogram raises obvious questions for the therapist that may be useful to the client to see in picture form as well, in order to become curious about other options for structuring the caregiving role(s).

When drawing a genogram with a caregiver, we always ask if there are people who are "like family" and how they function within the family. *Fictive kin* are persons outside of one's legally defined family who function as family (Chatters, Jayakody, & Taylor, 1994). Neighbors, members of a religious congregation, or coworkers can function as fictive kin. Fictive kin can be drawn on the genogram, even if they are not grafted onto the lines of the family tree. During health events, nonrelatives may function as family, and distant relatives may be pulled in closer to the care recipient than is typical for that family. In health settings, family therapists try to sort out who is in this health family (Rolland, 1994). CFT therapists need to understand who participates as family during health crises, chronic care phases, and beyond.

A fascinating aspect of CFT is the fact that information is often supplied in depth by one member of the family, reporting on relationship structures and dynamics. Obviously, a single source of information is always constrained by that person's perspective. Over time, a therapist gains a sense of the systematic biases of the caregiver that are likely to be influencing reports of the overall family system. A client with obvious narcissistic personality characteristics will inevitably report others as insufficiently attentive to his or her own needs. The therapist needs to hold the client's report as a piece of relevant but inconclusive data about how others actually interact. Over time, a client will describe others' behavior patterns and natural consequences of those patterns in the external world in ways that help the therapist make educated guesses about how others may view that person. Early in the assessment process, however, those biases are often not as evident, so a therapist needs to be cautious in adopting assumptions presented by a single source.

Triangulating information is a strategy used to address the limitations of a single reporter in family systems work as well as in qualitative research methods (Leech & Onwuegbuzie, 2007). In some cases, an independent report becomes available to add independent credibility to the caregiver's report. For example, a daughter caring for her father describes her mother as "having control issues." Later, a phone consultation with the client's sister elicits a similar description of their mother with an independent set of examples. Or the therapist receives a care plan from the facility where the father lives in which a concern is noted about the mother's frequent belligerent interactions with staff over their way of caring for him. Either of those independent sources of information validates the client's perspective.

Therapists will find the full genogram and analysis of family developmental history to be the contextual information needed to shape decisions about who will be involved in caregiving and in what ways. Initially, the focus is on who is providing what types of assistance and who is available to share the workload. Family members who are not involved in caregiving or supporting the caregiver may be relevant to engage in ways that are congruent with the overall family structure. Those who are cut off from the family will be very unlikely to engage in sharing the caregiving responsibility unless bridges are built to cross the cutoff chasm and resolve bitter feelings. On the other hand, members with viable relationships to the care recipient and/or caregiver but who are not now involved in care are potential people to engage.

WORKING WITH STRUCTURAL VARIATIONS

Every family structure has its challenges; there certainly is no right or normal or healthy structure that allows therapists to bypass consideration of how the family structure functions as a backdrop for caregiving. Therapists indeed are "inevitably ignorant" of each client family, and curiosity is the best strategy for figuring out the inevitable idiosyncratic complexities of each family. Although no particular family structure is bad, some structures are problematic during long-term caregiving phases because they constrain individual or family development. Acute health problems may be handled quite effectively within family patterns often associated with dysfunction, such as enmeshment (Rolland, 1994). In the context of long-term caregiving, family structures can be considered problematic when they interrupt the formation of effective decision making, communication, or emotional support. In other words, families need structures that support the individual development of members, and some structures make that very difficult.

Blatant structural problems are sometimes visible in a genogram depiction of a caregiving family. The presence of divorces and remarriages throughout multiple generations of a family suggests that there may be challenges in forming or maintaining intimacy bonds. Poor or ambiguous generational boundaries may be evident, as might occur when a wife is the legal decision maker for an impaired husband, and the absence of children leaves her unsure of whom to share that responsibility with as her own frailty increases. Genograms can depict cutoff relationships that functionally remove someone from the caregiving family or from at least part of that family if the person is cut off from some members but not others. Functional absence from the family is another condition of boundary ambiguity that stresses families (Boss & Greenberg, 1984). Functional absence may be due to missing-in-action status in a war, for example (Boss & Greenberg, 1984), or diminished capacity to participate fully, as in the case of dementia or brain injury (Boss, Caron, Horbal, & Mortimer, 1990). Structures need to have sufficient stability and connectedness to support individual members' attachments and to offer safe relationships that are present to provide love and basic resources.

Structural problems can occur simply because the family did not complete certain development tasks. For example, families that struggle to launch children tend to either hold them so close that development of basic adult independence is undermined or offer so little support that the emerging adult launches prematurely. The structures that result from incomplete or poorly handled developmental processes can affect caregiving (see the example in Exhibit 4.2). Two illustrative scenarios have presented in our clinical practices with surprising frequency: underdeveloped son caregivers who reside with aging mothers on whom they are financially dependent, and aging parents caring for an adult child with developmental disability. Although very different in terms of developmental processes, neither scenario offers aging parents a solid structure for care. Although long-term coresidence by members of multiple generations does not have to reflect a structural challenge, it is worth investigating the meaning and context when found in a genogram.

Family stories about the launching process during which children left home are often ripe with explanations for current conflicts, cutoffs, and enmeshments. Parents who had trouble letting go of their children may have inadvertently set up conditions that led the children to feel that they had to cut off the relationship in order to move into adulthood. Alternatively, the children may have felt they could not leave, setting up heavy involvement across generations that kept daughters in the middle of a conflicted parental marriage or positioned sons to divide time between family of origin and family of creation. Examples of

EXHIBIT 4.2

Dan

Dan has lived with his mother for 25 years in the family home, helping with odd chores between part-time jobs. He does not make enough money to pay for his own apartment, so he shares her house, paying for food for the two of them. He was shocked when the utilities were cut off last month after she neglected to pay the bills for several months. He knew she was having mild problems with memory, but why wouldn't she pay the bills?

clients' statements that suggest this type of structural challenge caused by family development difficulties include the following:

- "When I was 18, I knew I had to go, so I hopped a train and never looked back until I got the call from my sister that our mother was dying."
- "I was 15 when I had my first child, and my mother made sure I had what I needed; every time I left home after that I always ended up back with Mama to helped me pick up the pieces of the next failed marriage."
- "My husband's job took us to California but I couldn't stand being so far from home, so I came back to live with Mother and Daddy until he got his next assignment. When it was clear he would keep moving every 2 years, I begged him to give up that job but he wouldn't. So we divorced and I moved into my deceased grandmother's house where I still live, next door to my parents who help me with the kids."
- "I got into drugs for a while and ended up in prison, but got myself together enough to at least work part time. I just can't afford to live on my own yet so am still here in Mom and Dad's basement, which bugs my sisters but they just don't understand."

Family therapists have developed rich and useful theories and models that frame these problems in ways that can inform those who work with caregivers. The complex multigenerational histories of families can be the source of transmitted anxiety (Bowen, 1978), obligation, or unfinished equity issues that result in guilt (Boszormenyi-Nagy & Spark, 1984; Hargrave & Anderson, 1992). These may all distort emotion regulation within individuals or interpersonally. Lapses in family development tasks may complicate successive developmental tasks. Complicated or difficult transitions from stage to stage may establish fear or resistance to change. Learned patterns of communication or conflict resolution may constrain effective problem solving (Roberto, 1999).

Family history may also suggest dynamics and problems that complicate care for the older adult today. A daughter or son may have prematurely taken on a parental role while still in childhood if one parent was seriously ill, alcoholic, or deployed for long periods of time. The parentified role history may now be complicating caregiving as this person feels compelled to serve as primary caregiver regardless of current capability or the desire of other family members to share the burdens.

Aging parents with an adult child with a developmental or intellectual disability represent a special case of different launching or nonlaunching. Many in this current cohort of aging parents of adults with disability put extraordinary effort into protecting their sons and daughters from institutions in opposition to strong recommendations from their health care providers and family members in the 1950s or 1960s. The parents often maintained home-based care without support from formal services. As their own physiological aging compromises their functioning, the parents are forced to identify new options for launching their adult child with disabilities. Alternatively, premature aging of the adult with disabilities may reduce the supportive services provided to the aging parent that allowed the parent to remain at home. Disabilities systems are increasingly aware that parents' or adult children's age-related health crises can easily produce a dramatic crisis/transition for either or both (see the example in Exhibit 4.3).

Many, if not most, families have at least some adult member with significant psychopathology or personality disorder whose interpersonal style complicates communication about caregiving. A man with schizophrenia may have a strong emotional reaction to his mother's cancer and seek regular communication with family and health provider systems to express his worry. Communication with persons with emotional or psychological challenges may be disruptive to both primary caregivers and care recipients (see the example in Exhibit 4.4).

Particularly challenging are the social contexts that lack established rules for elder care, such as has occurred in recent decades in the sexual orientation minority community. Gay men, lesbians, transgendered, bisexual, and other sexually defined minorities have only recently established highly visible communities in which mutual support rules are being negotiated (Grossman, D'Augelli, & Dragowski, 2007). Previous underground support systems of care were necessary because of the exceptionally strong stigma against public identification with their sexual orientation. Those systems were not highly

EXHIBIT 4.3

David

David was overwhelmed by the sounds and activities of the emergency room where his mother, Beth, had been taken by ambulance after she had a stroke. He became increasingly agitated, and the ER staff were unable to take the time to manage his disruptive behaviors. David's mother was unable to provide directions to them because of the effects of her stroke, and yet she was terrified of what would happen to him while she was in the hospital. David's father sat helplessly in the waiting room, unable to assist David or his wife, because of his dementia. The disabilities agency was called to do an emergency placement for David into a group home. Beth's natural ambivalence about planning for her son's future ultimately led to him being placed in a home with strangers. Adult protective services was called to arrange an emergency placement for David's father, who could not live safely alone without assistance from his wife and son. When a second stroke took Beth's life 2 days later, neither David nor his father ever saw her or their home again.

EXHIBIT 4.4

Mr. Trujillo

Mr. Trujillo wants to divorce his wife of 45 years now that he is living separately from her in a senior housing facility, and his children support him. After his last surgery, the hospital discharge planner helped him identify assisted living as a residential alternative to going back home, where he would have to rely on his wife's very inconsistent care. His wife's bipolar disorder keeps her emotionally volatile as well, and although he feels a great deal of guilt about his decision, he is too tired to invest in keeping her stable. She is enraged that he is living separately and talking about divorce. She shows up regularly at his new assisted living home, and he is preparing to get a restraining order at the request of the facility.

visible, were rarely studied to understand their structures or operating rules, and were simply not available to many persons who needed them because of their relative invisibility. In the absence of a clear care system, competing care roles could hardly be addressed in any systematic way. What is one's responsibility to a long-term or short-term partner who requires full-time care but lacks insurance resources because he or she has never had the privilege of accessing health benefits as a domestic partner or spouse? How is the caregiver spouse to manage 24/7 care without financial resources to afford paid assistance, especially if the caregiver needs to work to support the household? There may be no one with whom to share responsibility if families have cut off contact because of negative biases about sexual orientation.

STARTING BEFORE YOU HAVE THE FULL PICTURE

How can a therapist begin intervention before gathering a deep and rich picture of family structure and function? Although we seek to obtain as much information as possible in the early interviews with caregivers, interventions usually must be initiated before all possible information can be gathered. Indeed, interventions generate useful information about family structure and function. In the early steps of CFT that focus on naming the problem, we have the opportunity to learn about family structures even while action is being initiated to gather information. The process of disseminating the findings from the naming step also tends to elicit structure information as the caregiver demonstrates enthusiasm or resistance to engaging members in particular roles. The greater scope of information is needed in cases in which caregivers do not function in their roles or engage family, as the therapist expected, or in which family conflict is a salient feature. Much of the broader family context information available to CFT therapists is shared incidentally as part of family stories or caregiving discussions.

TRACKING THE IMPACT OF STRUCTURAL CHALLENGES ON CAREGIVING

Structural characteristics of caregiving families set the stage for the dynamics of caregiving, and structural problems can provide extraordinary challenges to those in caregiving roles. A daughter acting as a caregiver for her mother with dementia and for her brother with disabilities will find it daunting to change living arrangements if their mutually symbiotic relationship means that a change for one forces a change for both. The dual task can seem overwhelming. Add any complexity into the family history and the care responsibilities may almost paralyze her. For example, if her brother abused her in the past, or if her other siblings had cut off their mother in anger over their deceased father's abuse of them during childhood, then she has added emotional and practical burdens in these responsibilities.

Clients initiating therapy are often in an immediate dilemma that requires a decision that they are hesitant to make because of the role implications. Many of our clients feel stuck about decisions because the very act of making a decision would initiate a role change. If family members strongly believe that a parent needs a medical evaluation, a driving test, or a move to more supportive housing, but the parent does not agree, then other family members may perceive themselves to be in a dilemma. Previous efforts to persuade the parent have not resulted in shared views or needed action. Any more direct involvement by the family reflects a very significant alteration in roles. Hence, family members feel stuck because they cannot tell for sure if it is time to make a major role transition.

Any transfer of decision-making authority from an older adult to anyone else without that person's explicit permission is a significant shift in family roles that has meaning to all involved. When a daughter acts on behalf of her mother by making an appointment her mother has refused to make, the daughter is announcing to self and others that she trusts her own judgment over her mother's so fully that she will intrude on her mother's autonomy. For anyone, that is a very meaningful transition in roles between the caregiver and care recipient, which is not likely to be done easily, without resistance, confusion, or angst. Families tend to try persuasion for a very long time before acting intrusively on an older family member's independence out of respect for historical roles. The legal right to make a decision for another requires a determination of incapacity, but most families navigate these transitions outside the legal arena. Ideally, families know ahead of time who is preferred by the care recipient to serve as proxy decision maker, and some type of durable power of attorney documents that preference. In cases of dementia, such documentation will ultimately be needed at the point at which formal providers get involved. Providers must have legal documentation of legal decision making authority for anyone other than the care recipient. Therapists will find it very helpful to become familiar with the processes for determining decision-making capacity and for invoking proxy decision makers (e.g., American Bar Association Commission on Law and Aging and American Psychological Association, 2005, 2006, 2008).

What gets in the way of family members trusting their judgment and stepping in when they know that an older adult is at risk? One reason the CFT model begins with a process of clarifying the problem is that family members need data to explain the older adult's failure to engage in good self-care and/or make decisions that are necessary to remain safe and independent. A strong evaluation provides the full picture that explains the problem to the older adult (unless cognitive impairment restricts ability to understand) and family in a framework that suggests possible solutions.

IDENTIFY THE CAREGIVING STRUCTURES

Families most commonly respond to significant care demands with a structure involving a primary caregiver and secondary caregivers (Stephens & Franks, 2009). In this structure, one person takes primary responsibility for making decisions and overseeing care needs. Other members may provide emotional support or practical support but recognize the primary caregiver's unique lead position. The selection of primary caregiver may not be explicit but is often assumed by one person whose previous roles make that position obvious. For example, spouses almost always assume the caregiving role if at all capable prior to consideration being given to any other family member (Stephens & Franks, 2009). If a spouse is unavailable or incapable, adult children are the next most likely caregivers for an older adult (Stephens & Franks, 2009). In-laws, particularly daughters-in-law, may be factored in as well. Siblings, nieces and nephews, and other family members, along with close friends, are other potential caregivers whose frequency of taking on the role is lower than children.

Secondary caregivers assist the primary caregiver with supports, ranging from finances, encouragement, help with solving difficult problems, or stepping in to provide respite that gives the primary caregiver a break. Secondary caregivers may not label the role for themselves explicitly, yet their roles are critical to sustaining the primary caregiver's capacity over time. The role structuring phase of CFT requires careful assessment of exactly who provides what support to the primary caregiver, in what forms, and how often.

Occasionally families fight over who will be the primary caregiver. In some cases, one person feels stuck with the role and engages in conflict with other family members who are perceived to be shirking their responsibility to function as the primary. Even if their role as primary caregiver is satisfactorily engaged, primary caregivers who report not feeling supported by secondary caregivers are at elevated risk of negative physical and mental health outcomes (Pinquart & Sörensen, 2005a, 2007). The demands on the primary caregiver are sufficiently difficult that support from others, both practical and emotional, makes a substantial difference. The specific behaviors leading to perceived support vary significantly across families, so the key is whether the primary caregiver feels supported and what it would take to ensure that perception of support.

Democracy is not a familiar structure in families across the life span and does not function well in caregiving (Fisher & Lieberman, 1996; Lieberman & Fisher, 1999). Perhaps only adult siblings whose parents have died are in a position to even attempt democracy, but realistically, siblings often have various reasons for not having equal footing in most decisions. Decisions involving parents almost always position one person to know more about the parents' well-being because of geographic nearness or involvement in health care or finances, or emotional closeness. Thus, democracy is unlikely to be a goal for family caregiving constellations involving multiple people; the primary-person-with-support structure is associated with greater success in managing the demands of caregiving. Of course, two people vying for the role as the primary caregiver also is not a stable caregiving structure. Families simply need to define a lead person with support surrounding from others.

The therapist can figure out the structure by asking the client to list all of the people who provide any level of assistance to the care recipient, offering several examples from the broad array of optional services. The people listed can then be linked to two visual maps to help make sense of role structures. First, the client may be asked to place those listed within concentric circles to represent the intensity of care services they provide (see Figure 4.2). Of course, the therapist needs to keep in mind that placement of persons within the circles is from the view of the client, a view that could be quite different from what another reporter would describe. This is an adaptation of the concentric circles task (Antonucci, 1986) used in social network analysis to query about the closeness of members of the social network of an individual. In this adaptation, the focus is on intensity of care provided. The innermost circle might be viewed as containing the primary caregivers, with secondary and even tertiary caregivers in the outer layers. The conversation during this task will have provided quite a bit of information about what each person actually does for the care recipient, which can be annotated on the figure. Follow-up questions can complete the information needed to understand who exactly is in the caregiving network and what exactly each person contributes. The therapist may recognize that a client is undervaluing or overvaluing the time and effort required to do a task by virtue of the placement within a circle that seems very inaccurate to the therapist. For example, a granddaughter who shops for groceries and cleans her grandmother's home each weekend would seem inappropriately placed in an outer circle. Be curious about those

FIGURE 4.2

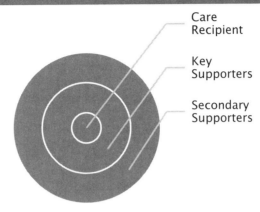

Care
Recipient

Key
Supporters

Secondary
Supporters

Concentric circles to identify caregiving support team.

apparent discrepancies in role definitions and valuing, because they may reflect ignorance or inattention to the demands of someone's role, or other family dynamics factors may be influencing the placement.

Caregiving annotations also can be added to the genogram, noting current and historical caregiving relationships. The historical context can be noted in responses to questions such as: Who provided care to previous generations? How was that determined within the family? Are there rules or themes in the caregiving relationships? How were care recipients treated within the family and how did their role shift as the illness progressed? What are the family stories and myths about caregiving from those earlier experiences?

Caregiving structures can be annotated with words, images, or color. A circle can be drawn around persons sharing a residence, for example. A circle might also be drawn around the primary and secondary caregivers to clarify who is in that circle of care. Conflicts about care may be depicted with a particular style or color of jagged line between the family members whose disagreements about care produce stress. Simply by highlighting a caregiver in color, patterns of distributing care roles within the family can become clearer. Additional notes about what services are provided by family members on the genogram link the caregiving information to other family structure information.

Following are key caregiving structure questions the therapist needs to be able to answer:

- If more than one person is involved, who is the primary caregiver? Who are the key secondary caregivers?
- What is the relationship of other caregivers to the primary? How does each provide support?
- What communication occurs regularly and intermittently?

EXHIBIT 4.5

Lisanne

Lisanne reports that she has one brother and two daughters and is married to a man who is also her business partner. Lisanne's father died 2 years ago, which precipitated her mother's move to live near her. By her report, Lisanne's brother is unwilling to help out with their mother's care because he was the primary caregiver for their father and views this as her turn. Lisanne's daughters both live out of state, available only for long weekend visits during which they try to help out with their grandmother as much as possible. She acknowledges she is doing too much, but her mother lacks finances to pay for home health providers to help her three times every day with medications (pills and insulin injections). Lisanne describes her husband as kind to her mother but not interested in becoming involved in hands-on care, a role he never even embraced as a father. He is frustrated, though, that Lisanne seems to be taking on so much for her mother. She agrees with the therapist's assessment that she needs more secondary caregiving help but can't figure out how to get it.

- Who is supportive of the well-being of the primary caregiver (regardless of whether this person is involved in care for the care recipient)?

The caregiving work needs to be distributed among individuals to ensure that each caregiver can sustain the load over time without undue cost to self or other responsibilities. If the list of tasks assigned to any one person is too long to be done within a normal lifestyle, or is too burdensome to be handled throughout a 24-hour period (see the example in Exhibit 4.5), the therapist may begin immediately to help the caregiver client seek assistance. Experience with caregivers over time is the basis for making these clinical judgments; no simple formula exists. Yet the overall pattern typically becomes clear. A primary caregiver with too much responsibility and no secondary helpers needs to begin working to build a team. On the other hand, broadly distributed tasks with no single person identified to be in charge likely signals a need for more organizational structure to ensure that someone is in charge when key decisions need to be made.

Structuring the Caregiver Roles

Caregiving structures work only if family members implement roles that are congruent with those family structures and the care recipient's needs. Aneshensel et al. (1995) positioned role implementation centrally within their metaphor of caregiving as a career. The career metaphor points to the importance of learning the role, implementing it, and unhooking from it when the needs of the care recipient position the caregiver in a new "job." We recognize five aspects of role enactment that must be in place for caregiving families to function well: role implementation, role clarity, role valuing, role identity, and management of role conflicts.

ROLE IMPLEMENTATION

Implementation refers to the pragmatics of the caregiving role(s), primarily supporting the activities of daily living (ADLs) and the instrumental activities of daily living (IADLs) needs of the care recipient. Assessment of role implementation involves a review of the ADL/IADL needs and noting how those are being met. Of course, some problem areas identified by the client will not necessarily have been addressed yet, suggesting gaps in the roles that need to be implemented. In most cases, however, some form of assistance will be in place, even if the family does not call it *caregiving*. Certainly, emotional support and less task-specific caregiving work needs to be addressed as well.

To help clarify the role activities, therapists may find it helpful to ask, "What are you doing for _____ now that you were not doing 10 or 20 years ago?" The contrast of *now* versus *then* can help families notice changes that have been so gradual they would not otherwise consider them noteworthy. Some role activity information was gathered naturally during the naming step when caregivers described their care recipient's symptoms and needs. Beliefs about the problem have been addressed in the first step on the intervention wheel. As described more thoroughly in Chapter 2, each client has a belief structure that frames the symptom or syndrome being described.

ROLE CLARITY

Family members benefit from being clear about role structures, regardless of what they are. Ambiguity does not serve families well, as demonstrated by a long line of research initiated by Pauline Boss and colleagues (Boss & Greenberg, 1984). Her work documents the stress on family members when roles are unclear because of the ambiguous status of a family member. Prisoners of war presented a significant dilemma to families whose lack of knowledge of the life or death status of a soldier during the Vietnam war left them stressed. A missing father, for example, left a significant hole in the family structure that could not be replaced legally, emotionally, or functionally, and yet his or her role activities had to be carried out by others in his absence. Boss et al. (1990) applied this construct of boundary ambiguity (is he in or out of the family?) to the experience of families dealing with dementia. The person with dementia is present, perhaps even engaging in some degree of family role participation, yet is so substantially changed in cognitive, emotional, and functional abilities that the family experiences a role ambiguity similar to that observed in families of prisoners of war.

Role clarity is perhaps most helpful in the arena of decision making within the family. Spouses or adult children of a person with cognitive impairment commonly struggle with the fear of usurping the dignity or personal authority of a loved one. Such fears can lead to avoidance of role clarity in order to avoid making decisions that could be distressing to the other person (see the example in Exhibit 4.6).

Even a person who embraces and identifies with a caregiving role may fail to implement the role because he or she is not clear on its parameters. Role clarity is achieved when the caregiver has an accurate understanding of the care recipient's problem (e.g., diagnosis), the level of support and care that is needed to balance autonomy and safety, and the caregiving role structures that can provide that care. Once needs are outlined as part of the naming step (see Chapter 2), roles must change in order for the caregiver to do his or her job, and those structural changes must be completed to the point of role clarity. Family members who understand their role and are clear about the parameters of the role are free to act without guilt, remorse, or the chronic confusion about whether they can or should act in key moments.

In contrast, ambiguous role boundaries almost guarantee conflict because family members lack a shared view of who should do what for whom under what circumstances. Poorly defined caregiving role boundaries are likely to lead caregivers to communicate ineffectively, with risks of mind reading, unspoken expectations, and disappointment that can spawn angry interchanges. In the absence of role clarity, family members can and will project their assumptions onto each other, leading almost inevitably to conflict over unmet expectations that easily yield perceptions of betrayal.

EXHIBIT 4.6

Karen

Karen tells you frankly that she knows her mother is a risk to the entire city when she heads out in her 1994 Lincoln Continental, which has been in three fender benders in the past 6 months that were her mother's fault. Karen has rescued her lost mother more times than she can count. Yet the thought of telling her mother she can't drive makes her sick. Karen does not want her mother to be sitting home alone feeling old and useless. Nor does she want to risk her mother's anger against her for restricting driving. So Karen avoids addressing the risks, abdicating a key component of her caregiver role. Karen is quite willing to engage the role actively and sacrificially as long as she is acting in accordance with her mother's wishes. But when caregiving requires her to protect her mother from risks that her mother does not recognize, Karen loses role clarity as well as courage. She insists that the idea of restricting driving is unfair to her mother, who should make her own decisions.

ROLE VALUING

Valuing different roles in families is one of the core challenges of family life from the earliest phase of family development, the formation of a partnership. Even prior to bringing another generation into the family, couples must work to accept the differences between them in how they accomplish the core tasks of relationship maintenance. Adding children often makes those differences even more salient. By the time families are decades old, the family tree is full of individuals with different gifts and challenges who are differentially valued by almost every other person on the family tree. Many adults live in the shadow of someone they feel was valued more, by self or others. Caregiving evolves within the contexts of these relationships so inevitably is caught up in the differential valuation of persons and their gifts.

A key question in caregiving families is whether the work of caregiving, the emotional toll, and the opportunities and challenges are valued. The caregiver himself or herself may not appreciate the scope of work being done or the emotional toll taken. Valuing of caregiving begins with acknowledgement of the magnitude of the role, including the work, emotions, relationship shifts required, financial and other costs, and the impact on self and others. Until the caregiving role is valued, no realistic restructuring can take place.

ROLE IDENTITY

What exactly does it mean to say one is a *caregiver*? The range of caregiving work accomplished by persons self-identifying as caregivers is remarkable. On average, caregivers provide 20.4 hours per week of care, with those living with the care recipient providing 39.3 hours per week (National Alliance for Caregiving, 2009). For some, a phone call to support another's work is an act of caregiving that costs little, whereas that call might weigh heavily on the emotions of another. Caregivers who devote several hours per day or who are in the role 24/7 have a different meaning to adopting the term *caregiver* as a role identified with the self.

During the course of a chronic condition, caregivers often experience significant changes in role identity. A spouse who begins serving as caregiver to a person with dementia may engage in a few isolated role changes early on (e.g., taking over bill paying, arranging to eat out more often to reduce the burden of meal preparation). Later, that spouse may take on more substantive roles of medication management or structuring daily activities and prompting self-care tasks such as bathing. A few years later, the caregiving spouse may be serving as advocate within a residential dementia care environment, interpreting the care recipient's personal history and preferences to a staff who knows nothing about the person. Each of these role shifts involves learning new tasks, but it also involves rewriting the role identity associated with caregiver.

Discrepancies between role responsibilities and identification with the caregiver role are a source of distress for caregivers (Montgomery & Kosloski, 2011). Family members need to maintain an accurate understanding of their own internalized norms along with the actual caregiving role tasks being accomplished, with opportunities to review and revise either to keep them aligned. Self-appraisals of failure to achieve personal role standards, even if they are highly inappropriate expectations, can lead to distress. In essence, caregivers can get in trouble if they do not recognize the load they are carrying, if they assign themselves tasks that are inconsistent with the needs of the care recipient or that exceed their capabilities, or if they use inappropriate standards as a basis for appraising performance as successful or not (see the example in Exhibit 4.7).

A key question is how the caregiver(s) have integrated the role into their own self-identity. Discrepancies between identity and role performance or expectations are likely to lead to personal or interpersonal distress. To what extent does the client identify as a caregiver, and how does the self-identification map onto a realistic description of his or her role? Every family member who provides care does not need to apply that word to his or her role, of course. But ignoring the caregiving role is not healthy either, because the role is associated with feelings, actions, and thoughts that are organized around its work and identity. Those ignoring the role are often ignoring the scope of its impact on their lives and the scope of its impact on the care recipient. In our experience, caregivers who seek help are rarely overinvolved but commonly are doing less than is truly needed by the care recipient and crediting themselves less with the size and shape of their caregiving roles. Obviously, the opposite exists as well: families who err in overstating the scope and personal identity of the role for what appear to be self-serving reasons. Therapists need to be aware of the range of possibilities for making errors in role identification. Discrepancies of role performance or role identification from the tasks needed to support the care recipient adequately are all key components of role identity analysis.

Hesitancy to embrace the role of caregiver is likely to be problematic if the role identity far understates the care recipient's need for care.

EXHIBIT 4.7

George

George visits his wife daily at the care facility where she resides, often pitching in to provide some of her care when the staff is busy. He may toilet her, transfer her to bed, change her clothing, administer therapeutic foot cream, empty her catheter, or feed her. These are all tasks familiar to him as caregiver. He finds it much more challenging to seek staff assistance to do those care tasks; advocacy and care management are new role identities that are less comfortable than providing the direct care tasks himself.

Misalignment in role identity and the caregiver role that is needed predicts a poor outcome for either caregiver or care recipient, so efforts need to be initiated to align the role identity with the role demands.

Key role identity questions include the following:

- How accurately does the caregiver understand the work he or she is doing for the care recipient?
- Does he or she discount the work done, ignoring its value or impact?
- Does he or she overvalue the role, ignoring the apparent capabilities of the care recipient or the contributions of other caregivers?

MANAGEMENT OF ROLE CONFLICT

When family members disagree about care strategies, CFT therapists need to ask whether the disagreeing parties have a similar base of information available to them. Many role disagreements are caused by differential knowledge or understanding of the problem. We emphasize the importance of disseminating the name for the problem (diagnoses, etiology, functional assessment, treatment plans) for this very reason. Family members who have different understandings of the problems faced by the care recipient and primary caregiver are highly likely to generate divergent ideas about how to provide care. After information has been disseminated and discussed, the family still may need help talking through care strategies, but many families have existing communication and problem-solving skills that are sufficient for them to proceed without additional assistance.

The second focus for careful consideration with conflicted families is values. We notice that conflict among family members often starts around care strategies and deteriorates into a blaming match in which dispositional attributions about each person's personality or character are used to explain the differences in strategy preference. For example, siblings who differ on whether to care for a mother with dementia in her own home or move her to assisted living may quickly shift focus to the motives they believe underlie those choices. "You just don't want to spend Mom's money so you can be sure you inherit more, even if it means she is sitting alone in her house every day." "Well, you just don't want to be bothered with the time and energy it takes to keep her in her own home." Therapists need to direct these siblings away from the personal accusations about motivations and character to reframe the issue as a choice among strategies. The deep hurts from earlier life that are unresolved, and perhaps unresolvable, can't be addressed during CFT, so the therapist needs to insert a more positive possibility into the family that they may actually share several values related to caring for their loved ones. Later in this chapter we offer specific strategies for helping families examine their values about balancing autonomy and safety, which lie at the heart of many of these conflicts.

Old structures within the family are made visible or become salient when long-term conflicted families face the challenges of caring for an older member. These long-term, deep divides are unlikely to be resolved at a time of high demand and high anxiety on the family, so CFT directs the family away from the hospital, residential care facility, or primary care office as a venue for exploring their differences. Instead, CFT becomes more narrowly focused on the specific conditions for care that need to be met and on a specific plan for delivering that care. Warring siblings or tense parent–child relations may be unresolvable, but they can be sent to the background in favor of a focus on exactly what the older adult needs at this moment. Some of the greatest strains on staff in residential facilities come from conflicted families who use the older adult resident as the flashpoint or pawn in the ongoing conflict. Siblings may compete to be in control of care or may attempt to outdo one another in vying for attention from the elder or from staff. Staff may not be able to do anything right in everyone's eyes, being forced to choose whose directives to follow in the nuances of care. Residential facilities and other care agencies may be forced to establish visiting schedules or communication channels to which family members are limited in order to protect care staff from being caught in the middle of an impossible situation.

Family Caregiving Dynamics

Although a genogram is a static snapshot of structures, caregiving structures and roles need to be understood as dynamic structures that respond to particular needs. Knowing who does what today is a great first step, but information about change over time is also important to understand. Indeed, the ways in which caregiving roles shift over time are relevant to understanding the adaptation process that will be the core work of therapy.

Dynamics are the processes by which family systems respond to change or input. In the case of caregiving families, the focus of attention is usually on changes in the care recipient but needs to extend to changes in lives of other members as well. How are the primary caregivers noticing change and responding to it? How are secondary caregivers and other family members learning about those changes and about the new care structures implemented by the primary caregiver? What other relationship dynamics are influencing these communications within the care system? Outside of caregiving, how do the members of this role structure interact?

Dynamics information is gathered over time, from a combination of client reports and the therapist's observation of what occurs when families change an interaction pattern. Certainly, the caregiver client is likely to report on family dynamics in the context of describing the caregiving situation. Some caregivers bring in e-mails, letters, or reports of oral conversations that exemplify interactions among family members. Others can be prompted to try an interaction as part of an intervention (e.g., to solicit more supportive assistance), to which there are likely to be reactions that illustrate the family dynamics.

Of course, a single source of information can be biased, and the potential for such biases needs to be considered carefully. This style of reasoning about the family system relies on clients to reveal their biases over time in the narratives they tell. Careful analysis of the described behavior of others, combined with a description of responses to those behaviors in the environment, provides a form of independent information to the therapist (see the example in Exhibit 4.8). When a mother describes her caregiver son as a "horrible son," yet the facts about his life suggest that he is well loved by the world, stable in relationships and work, and happy in daily life, the therapist needs to question the mother's frame. In this case, the triangulation process used to validate a single perspective leads the therapist to hypothesize that the caregiver son is in fact a reasonable person whose behaviors toward the client are good faith efforts to address difficult situations even though they fail to meet the mother's desires or needs. Without a direct source of data, therapists need to be cautiously aware that they are dealing only with hypotheses. Yet therapeutic hypotheses about family interactions that cannot be witnessed directly form a basis for choosing intervention strategies that may in fact test the assumptions embedded in the hypotheses.

An ideal situation for CFT work with difficult families is to witness the dynamics in person. Therapists may be able to engage other family members to participate in session(s), even when the help-seeking caregiver does not believe others would attend. Indeed, inviting other mem-

---

EXHIBIT 4.8

Patricia

Patricia describes her family members primarily in terms of what they do or fail to do for her. The therapist realizes that Patricia's style is highly self-referential in ways that suggest narcissistic traits so is naturally suspicious that Patricia's children may not be as bad as her descriptions suggest. The genogram shows that there is no evidence of interpersonal conflict among the siblings and that each adult child is in a long-term relationship with a spouse or partner, has children, and has a long-term stable employment history. The therapist asks Patricia about specific examples of interaction among the siblings and between each adult child and his or her partner/spouse. Patricia describes normal conflicts and family struggles but nothing as dramatic or harsh as the description of their failures with her. The therapist hypothesizes that Patricia has, or can obtain, more support from the children than she perceives them offering. Only Patricia's biased perspective limits what the relationships can offer her.

bers to participate in the therapy, whether for a single session or for the entire therapy, provides an ideal way for the therapist to gather independent data on family dynamics. Assuming one family member initiated CFT, the therapist may immediately ask that person to invite others to join the therapy or may be more strategic about preparing for other(s) to participate for a more specific purpose. The process by which that person approaches the invitation and participation of others is informative. How did the communication happen (e-mail, phone, in person)? What exactly was the request? What rationale was provided? What were the responses? How hard was it to schedule the family session? Who seemed most invested? Who served as troubleshooter for challenges in scheduling?

Any opportunity to witness multiple family members interact provides a wealth of information about the family dynamics over which caregiving is now layered. For example, when a son did not believe his sister's report of their mother's enhanced dramatic acting out behavior, the son came to town to visit the family, during which time a therapy session was scheduled. Direct observation of the dynamics between the siblings provided the therapist with invaluable information to use in coaching communication options. In some cases, the CFT therapist primarily witnesses family interactions in e-mails and can coach family members in responding carefully (see Figure 4.3 and the example in Exhibit 4.9).

FIGURE 4.3

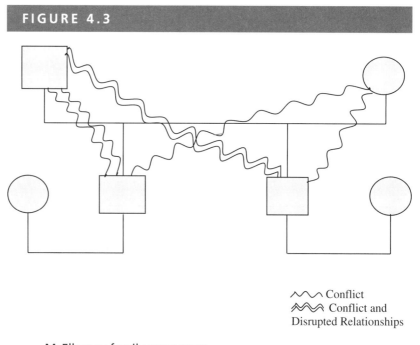

∿∿∿ Conflict
≈≈≈ Conflict and
Disrupted Relationships

McElhaney family genogram.

EXHIBIT 4.9

Mrs. McElhaney

Mrs. McElhaney wanted her sons, who lived at a distance, to be more supportive of her care for Mr. McElhaney, a man with frontal-temporal dementia whose impulsivity and difficult behaviors were very hard to manage. She reported to the therapist that the sons were quite resistant to coming to visit in the next few months. Although they cited heavy work schedules, she believed they were mainly hesitant to increase their involvement with their father who had a history as a harsh, distant father. The therapist helped Mrs. McElhaney depict these relationships in a genogram (Figure 4.3). Although unwilling to visit the parents, their son, who was an academic physician in a major research institution 1,500 miles away, invited his parents to visit him and had a plan for his father to be reevaluated in the geriatric neurology unit at his university hospital. The son was clearly skeptical about the diagnosis and requested a copy of the neuropsychological evaluation along with the evaluator's curriculum vitae. Although the neuropsychologists' training was outstanding, the son insisted to his mother that professionals at his institution could provide superior information about Mr. McElhaney's problem. The son also treated his mother's descriptions of intense, impulsive behaviors as overly dramatized accounts that reflected distortions because of her personality disorder.

The CFT therapist primarily witnessed those interactions in e-mails and coached Mrs. McElhaney in responding carefully to the emotionally charged missives. The therapist recognized and validated the son's insistence on personal control over his area of expertise (i.e., health care) and strongly encouraged Mrs. McElhaney to arrange the trip. The therapist recognized that Mrs. McElhaney truly needed her sons' support, and neither son would accept the diagnosis until a second opinion was obtained from a source trusted by the expert son. Furthermore, the visit would provide a personal experience with the father's behavior in the son's home that was likely to help him gain perspective on his mother's daily experience that he had discounted.

Indeed, the trip worked as hoped. The second opinion affirmed the diagnosis. The son and his family gained a profound appreciation of Mr. McElhaney's daily behavior problems. Although hesitant to support their mother's concerns without questioning whether her personality was making it more dramatic than needed, the sons were not blatantly discounting of her challenges in caring for their father. They supported her in subsequent decisions to add professional help, despite their father's rage, and her later decision to place him in a residential facility.

Information about caregiving dynamics that have been examined within the context of broader family dynamics paints a picture of where changes might be possible. The communication patterns, including verbal interchanges as well as behavior toward each other, are the explicit data from which family dynamics are analyzed. The CFT therapist integrates observations of dynamics to form working hypotheses about how particular people will respond to particular communications from specific other members of the family. Because interactions tend to be redundant within families, past interaction patterns form a basis for predicting future ones. Interventions are designed to interrupt those patterns by introducing novelty. The therapist should form a working hypothesis about which new interactions are most likely to result in a positive outcome (e.g., a family member engaging in a new way, someone offering additional assistance to the primary caregiver) before attempting an intervention. Tight scripting of novel interactions is not possible, but general predictions about opportunities for change are the foundation of family system interventions.

The cumulative effort to integrate information about family structure, family developmental history, family dynamics, and the caregivers' roles is a weighty clinical task. CFT therapists are often flooded by information that does not reduce to simple diagnostic statements. Across sessions the therapist builds an ever-expanding database of family information that shapes hypotheses about how to structure roles for the best outcomes for caregiver, care recipient, and other family members.

Simplistically, the therapist wants to determine whether the caregiving role structures are adequate to meet the care recipient's needs (are there enough services provided to support any behavioral deficits?), are structured in a way that does not overly burden a single individual, are structured to build strong support for the primary caregiver, and are structured in a way that supports clear role identity. Discrepancies between what is needed and what is being performed must be addressed by reconfiguring roles to add services where they are needed. Formal as well as informal caregivers may be part of the solution to a problem of inadequate services. On the other hand, excessive role involvement by families can generate excess disability in care recipients, leading to added health and mental health problems and premature mortality. The CFT therapist must understand how to assess misalignment of role performance with caregiving needs. Understanding of the dynamics used by a particular family to restructure roles is also foundational to interventions that may be needed to redistribute role responsibilities.

Reconfiguring Roles: Principles to Guide Interventions

When the picture becomes clear as to what the older adult care recipient needs from the family, what services the family currently provides, and how roles are structured to offer the care, the therapist and client can map care needs onto that picture. Equally important, caregiving structures that are unsustainable also become evident (e.g., highly burdened primary caregiver, overinvolved siblings, distant underinvolved children). Therapists begin the slow process of experimenting with family structural and role changes. The remainder of this chapter describes principles and strategies to implement them that we use to guide efforts to reorganize family caregiving roles. We recognize that therapists are infinitely creative in building interventions for families, so here we state core values and principles to guide them. The cases in Chapter 8 illustrate two family's solutions to restructuring.

ACTIVELY FACILITATE ROLE TRANSITIONS

Therapists may use multiple strategies for facilitating role transitions within families. The following list includes several approaches we have found helpful within CFT practice: clarifying values among family members; enhancing urgency when risk for the care recipient is high; building on successes; modeling language within sessions; and, ultimately, creating new family structures.

Clarify Values

CFT presumes that many of life's powerful values are embedded in polarities that maintain a tension between competing poles in order to keep from tipping all of the way in one direction or the other. Examples include the inherent tension between individualism and collectivism, aloneness and togetherness, as well as autonomy and safety, which were described previously. Marital fights often have these values dilemmas at their core. "Can I buy the sailboat, or do I save for the children's college expenses" can be viewed as a dilemma between individualism and collectivism. "Do we let Mom live out her last years at home, knowing she is at risk for falling or require her to move into a residential care facility that affords her less independence than she wants?" Many family conflicts are simply polarizations of these alternative values between people. One person ends up voicing only one side and another person voices the other side of the dilemma. In reality, both persons probably value both ends of the dilemma.

One way to ensure that such dilemmas remain located in the inevitable values tensions that all share, rather than becoming ossified in an interpersonal conflict, is to engage each person in stating his or her values. A simple exercise for eliciting values statements is described here:

> We need to talk soon about how you all want to provide care to your father, but I find it helpful to wait to discuss the *how* until we have discussed the *why*. So I would like to take a few minutes to talk about what is important to you about your father's life between today and the day he dies. First, what do you want most for him as he lives his last years? Then, what would you hope for his dying to be like?

Almost all family members will say some kind of statement that contains three messages: Each person will want him (a) to be as independent as possible for as long as possible, (b) to be safe so he doesn't experience a frightening trauma (e.g., falling and being incapacitated while alone in a house that no one checks for days), and (c) to die without trauma or drawn out painful conditions that require institutional care. Each person will use different words and likely speak longer and more vehemently about one of those points than another. But when the sharing is complete, it is almost always possible for the therapist to say something like the following:

> As I listen to you, I am struck by the fact that you all want your father to experience maximum autonomy or independence possible while being safe, and that you wish for him a peaceful non-traumatic noninstitutional dying process. Does that sound right?

Once affirmed (or potentially corrected, although rarely does anyone discount one of those culturally sanctioned values), a therapist can then help the family note that although they share values, there are variations in how they voice the values:

> I also notice that each of you finds it easier to state some of those points than others. I notice that some of you are highly sensitized to the issue of autonomy (or independence) and automatically notice when it might be at risk. Others of you are highly sensitized to issues of safety and are quick to notice risk. If I were to guess, based on my experience with you today, I would guess that _____ is the quickest and perhaps even most passionate voice for autonomy, whereas _____ is the quickest and perhaps most passionate voice for safety. Does that ring true for you?
>
> I also want to notice that all of you stated that you value both autonomy and safety. You just have personalities and life experience that position you to notice and respond a bit more to one of those than the other. So I predict that when we begin to talk about care strategies, you will follow those proclivities and find it easier to lean toward strategies that line up with the value that is most top-of-mind for you. That can be really useful as we talk about the very difficult choices that lie ahead of you. We can be sure that _____ will notice when we begin to shift away from autonomy, even a little bit, toward the safety side of this balancing act. And likewise, _____ is likely to be the first to notice when we shift toward safety at some cost to autonomy. This will be very helpful to us. I invite and encourage you to speak your mind when you notice the balance seems to be tipping. We all want to keep both of these values in mind as we proceed to plan for care of your father.

A values discussion such as this one, followed by the invitation for people to share their biases that are useful to keep the conversation balanced, goes a long way toward keeping the values dilemma visible without embedding it in interpersonal conflict. In other words, this conversation reduced the interpersonal struggle involved in the balancing process. Valuing difference rather than viewing it as harmful is a key step in launching an open conversation. The therapist is also now positioned to compliment biases as informative, relieving the family from having to resolve decades-old tensions between different personalities and biases that have played out in many, many interpersonal conflicts. At this moment, the long interpersonal history is a fact that needs to be neutralized as much as possible in favor of focusing on the older adult care task of the moment.

Enhance Urgency When Risk is High

Role changes are hard to implement, and family members often view them as impossible. Yet, a simple shift in the premises made by the family opens doors to new possibilities. A common example we encounter in the early work on naming the problem is that an older adult may resist going to a professional for evaluation (e.g., physician, neuropsychologist, driving school). The family member seeking help often states this resistance in the form of "she just won't go, and there is nothing I can do to make her." More elaborate forms of the protest may include, "I can't very well carry her to the car, and short of that, she is just refusing to go." The premise here is that the older adult's willful refusal is the final word. No persuasion efforts have altered the refusal, and thus there is no option to make her go. If, however, we shift the premise from the assumption that the family's job is to persuade her to go, then the family actually knows how to make action happen. The therapist can enhance the sense of urgency by saying something like the following:

> If you found your mother on the floor of her home when you arrived, with a weak right arm and leg and slurred incoherent speech, how would you respond to your mother's statement that you *must not* call the ambulance?

Every family with whom we have worked has quickly noted that they would bypass their mother's wishes and call the ambulance. When we inquire what makes them comfortable acting against her wishes in that circumstance, they note that the situation is obviously a health crisis and not calling would leave her vulnerable to deteriorating health or death. At this point, we observe that it is interesting that they actually know how to bypass her wishes, but that in the current circumstance they are not willing to do so. Risk and urgency seem to be the distinguishing characteristic of our little imagery exercise that allowed the family to act.

Risk and urgency are almost always present in the circumstance that provoked the family to seek assistance, so we are easily able to point those out. Once we have reviewed the current situation's equivalent of the stroke image in the exercise, we usually have a better basis for brainstorming options for moving beyond persuasion as a strategy for getting the assessment needed.

The impact of an exercise such as this is similar to being stunned by being hit by the proverbial 2 × 4, which produces insight. The exercise is particularly helpful with people who have previously been stuck in resistance to action that in effect would move them into new roles. We have affectionately "hit them up the side of the head" to get attention and leverage for looking together for new strategies for creating change. At times, a 2 × 4 won't do the job, and we look for a 2 × 6, or more intensive strategies to create urgency to act in the face of growing risk.

Spouses are often entrenched in a role structure that disallows one person to decide for another. Couples may have a long history of collaborating on decisions, such that even as one member of the couple loses cognitive abilities, the other member insists on achieving consensus in all decisions. For older adults whose dementia-induced anosognosia makes it impossible for them to view risk realistically, the well spouse is effectively impotent to create good decisions consensually but has growing anxiety about safety risks. In such cases, the therapists can enhance the sense of urgency by saying something like the following:

> Imagine you have just awakened in a hospital intensive care unit, having just survived a heart attack and stroke. Others can't understand your speech, and indeed you aren't sure you are even talking out loud. In your head, you are screaming to the staff to check on your husband who is at home. Of course, they do not know that he is alone, waiting for you to return from an errand he can't recall, incapable of acting on his own to prepare food, take medications, or prepare to go to bed. But wait a minute—how many hours have you been here? What day is it? What if he went a whole day without his insulin?

A chronic challenge in CFT is getting family caregivers to create plans and safety nets of services that would keep this terrifying scenario from happening. Instead of recognizing that every day is a series of risky situations in which changes in the caregiver's health and well-being could render the care recipient 100% vulnerable, caregivers often make vague references to being hardy or resilient, as if they were immortal. We notice that efforts to persuade them to look at the risks logically are far less effective than this type of an imagery exercise that makes the risks salient. Once motivated, the caregiver can be guided through the role shift from solo-invincible-caregiver to a role as advocate and case manager of a range of services that have redundancy built in to address any changes in his or her ability to meet the care recipient's needs.

Occasionally, we use strategies designed to generate almost intolerable urgency in situations in which failure to shift roles is creating unacceptable risks.

> I would like to discuss a difficult topic with you because I think it will help us figure out your priorities. What is most important to you about how you want your mother to die?

Or as an alternative,

> I want you to imagine that you just got a call from the morgue that your mother's body is being transferred there from the hospital emergency room where she was treated unsuccessfully after being found alone and in pain on the floor of her apartment after a fall. You have been so worried about her consistent resistance to moving into assisted living that you have forgotten that you are living every hour of every day with a very real risk of getting that call from the morgue. Although she cannot understand it, she is highly likely to be happily engaged in social activities every single day in assisted living. You are letting her inability to see what lies in the future that is good leave her at high risk of dying in a way you and she both would consider horrible.

Build on Successes

Helping families notice variability in behavior opens up possibilities. Family members are highly likely to notice one another's tendencies that are persistent and steady over time, missing the variability in behavior that provides a clue about how to create change. "She always" or "he never" statements stop creative problem solving before it has started. Yet when did something work well? What were the circumstances? Specific details are needed regarding the environmental contexts, time of day, who was involved, exactly what happened, and how the desirable scenario unfolded. Once detailed, the family and therapist often can see that the desired behavior is possible, under certain circumstances. The behavior may not occur often, or when everyone wishes it, but if it can occur, then there is hope for replicating that occurrence deliberately (see the example in Exhibit 4.10).

This strategy pushes against the family's urge for homeostasis in following family rules. *Family rules* are summary statements of how interactions typically unfold or are expected to unfold. Observers are often able to state these rules after a fairly brief period of observation because the family follows them so faithfully. Family members are usually not consciously considering the rule while they interact but are merely following familiar behavioral patterns as if the unspoken rules were guiding their behavior. For example, Sally quickly intercedes when her brother is critical of their mother, almost as if there is a rule dictating the behavior sequence. John's jaw tenses when Peter begins to speak. Larry jumps to fill Jane's glass before it becomes empty. Tanner and Philipa fight after sex.

Efforts to interrupt familiar behavior sequences usually meet with considerable resistance. Systems attempt to maintain stability in the interactive movement among parts, a process termed *homeostasis*. A commonly used metaphor for family homeostatic mechanisms is a household thermostat that acts to maintain temperature within a predefined range. The thermostat notices when temperature in the room

---

EXHIBIT 4.10

Milt

Milt and his sisters, Fanny and Carolyn, were stymied by their parents' refusal to even discuss moving from the big farm house 30 miles from town, despite the fact that their mother now needed dialysis several times a week at the medical center in town. All three of the children had broached the topic in the past month but gotten nowhere. Dad just put his foot down, and Mother was too passive to protest. The therapist asked the siblings which one of them had the longest conversation. Fanny had actually discussed the challenge of traveling for dialysis with her parents for 20 minutes or more, which was four times the length of conversations the other two had generated. Fanny's conversation was outlined in detail, which led the siblings to recognize that she had not attempted to discuss moving, only the challenge of transportation several times each week. Her conversation had yielded a discussion of getting an apartment in town, however, which was far more than the other two could get the parents to consider. The therapist built on the details of Fanny's approach to outline the next intended conversation. Apparently the parents could recognize the practical challenges of traveling to town multiple times each week, despite their deep connection to their home in the country, and were worried about how that would be possible in bad weather, which led them to brainstorm about options for being in town part of the week. The siblings believed that the suggestion to move was possible because of Fanny's approach, so they began to plan a shared conversation with the parents that used the same principles.

---

is out of the range defined as acceptable and triggers a heater to blow warm air until the temperature is back in range. So in families, familiar patterns of behavior function to maintain the emotional climate in the relationships within a particular range that is desirable, tolerable, and/ or familiar (even if not desirable). The urge for homeostasis is powerful, leading family members to resist change from the familiar.

CFT therapists need to find examples of behaviors that occurred outside the familiar patterns or sequences in order to open the family to true role changes. Family therapy models emphasize the importance of perturbing or interfering with familiar patterns sufficiently that new ones can emerge. The possibility is that the new ones will be more adaptive for the current circumstance than the former, long-term behavior sequences. Thus, therapists will find it valuable to look for the instance in the past in which the desired behavior or outcome occurred and attempt to perturb the family system (i.e., break the rules) sufficiently to allow new patterns to emerge (see the example in Exhibit 4.11).

Model Language

Role change is about communicating differently in words and behaviors. The redundancy in family patterns that is described previously interferes with experimentation with novelty. Family members cannot figure out what to say differently from what they have always said.

EXHIBIT 4.11

Kayleigh

Kayleigh's mother refused to see the doctor. The therapist investigated instances in which Kayleigh's mother had actually gone ahead and done something that she had verbally refused to do. Kayleigh recognized that, indeed, her mother had gone to the dentist when Kayleigh simply made the appointment for her mother at the same time she made appointments for other family members. Although the mother complained bitterly, she went to the dentist for a checkup and was grateful afterward. The therapist helped Kayleigh notice the steps in the behavior sequence that seemed to work, steps that in fact implied different roles for Kayleigh and her mother.

In the sequences that led to her mother refusing doctor appointments, Kayleigh was encouraging her mother to make the appointment. In the dental example, Kayleigh made the appointment and announced to her mother that she would pick her up to take her when she took the children. Kayleigh responded to her mother's complaints with a calm, quiet voice: "I'm sorry you don't want to go, Mother, but you really need to protect your teeth, and so I've made the appointment and will be by to pick you up on Thursday at 2:30." Kayleigh did not attempt to defend her choice to make the appointment or persuade her mother about its value. She simply stated the facts and expectations. Her mother responded by being ready to go when Kayleigh arrived to take her to the appointment. Kayleigh and her therapist spent time exploring Kayleigh's previous ambivalence about taking over a task that her mother could previously accomplish on her own. Kayleigh acknowledged that it was painful to accept that her mother was no longer independent.

Therapists need to offer new language options and often need to role-play in order for families to gain experience actually saying these new statements (see the example in Exhibit 4.12).

Opportunities to coach a client through new ways of communicating are the essence of role change. Communication includes behavior as well as language. Some caregivers need to learn to walk away from an intense situation without speaking, after which the care recipient shifts focus to a more compliant stance with the caregiver. Others need to learn new language. Still other caregivers need mainly to learn to say statements without invoking a defensive tone of voice. Therapists need to help identify new communications and coach the family through those new options until the family has a sense of efficacy in implementing the new behaviors or language.

Create New Family Structures

Older adults and families often seek a face-saving solution that allows the care recipient to view himself or herself as a person with dignity in managing personal affairs, even when impairments limit capacity for full independence. CFT encourages families to be creative in this sensitive matter of labeling roles. Being known as a care recipient or a

---

EXHIBIT 4.12

Laura

Laura could not figure out how to discuss finances with her father. He had never shared financial information with her or anyone else. Recently, it became clear that he was not handling personal bill paying effectively, even with a subtle prompting system she set up to remind him to check the bill cubbyhole twice a month. Evaluations documented that he had dementia of moderate intensity, so his difficulties made sense and were unlikely to improve. Multiple professionals agreed that Laura needed to take charge of his personal financial responsibilities, leaving him with a fund-limited checkbook and credit card that allowed him to maintain access to funds, albeit limited. Laura could not figure out how to talk to him about the need for her to take over the regular bills. Her guilt about going against his wishes was overwhelming.

The therapist role-played with her, taking the role of Laura and letting Laura play her father. After several role-plays, they had created together several statements for Laura to say and switched roles. Laura was then able to role-play with her taking the role of herself, and she felt far more prepared to have an actual conversation with her father. The following week she reported that the conversation with him had followed a path they didn't anticipate, but she had many options for handling it and so was able to complete the agreement with him for her to manage his main finances. Although she was concerned about the changing dynamics in their relationship, she noted to her therapist that she would have felt much worse if her father's assets had been lost because she had not stepped in to help.

---

caregiver undermines dignity for some families. A 90-year-old retired stockbroker may not want his son taking over finances, even if he recognizes that he is struggling to see the small print or track the large level of detail in his complex portfolio. Vision impairment renders Helen unable to read bank statements, but she wants to be in charge of all decisions about her finances and to keep them private from her children. Innovative role structures are needed.

One model that has worked in our clinic is to ask an older adult to select people to serve as their personal "staff." Sometimes one person is selected; other situations call for a committee. One option for accomplishing this is to invite the care recipient to identify members who could serve on committees to implement the values and intentions of the care recipient. In other words, the care recipient is in charge of saying what he or she wants to happen and determining who will make it happen (see the example in Exhibit 4.13).

Rapid decisions may need to be made in a high-risk situation. If the person's cognitive impairment limits his or her ability to recognize the problem or contribute to the problem solving of alternative solutions, family members will be forced to implement a decision coercively. Bypassing the older adult's protests that assistance is not needed, family members will implement a decision unilaterally, as long as appropriate legal documents are in place to support their right to do so. On the other hand, therapists may need to confront the adult children's overwhelm-

---

EXHIBIT 4.13

Mr. and Mrs. Vitaliano

Mr. and Mrs. Vitaliano both showed signs of cognitive impairment but retained capacity to be in charge of many aspects of their own lives. Complex spreadsheets outlining their projected assets over time were overwhelming to both of them, however. They appointed a finance committee consisting of their accountant, one son who lives at a distance, and a local long-term trusted friend. The CFT therapist helped them assign this committee the tasks of maximizing assets and telling the couple when financial decisions were looming. The committee met with the Vitalianos to review the trends (rather than the details) and discuss the values by which the next set of decisions would be made.

---

ing fears that are driving them to put excessive safety measures in place for a parent who does not really require them. Family members may have trouble tolerating risk and behave in overly protective ways that they have no legal right to impose on the older adult.

Decisions made in the earlier stages of caregiving (through mutual discussions between caregiver and care recipient) can help the caregiver during later stages know that he or she is following the values and wishes of the care recipient as stated when the care recipient was capable of processing the information and offering an opinion. Values questionnaires are another way older adults can provide comfort to family members who must make decisions on their behalf. More information about the older adult's preferences is almost always better to support the legality of a proxy's decision as well as the sense of moral responsibility that others have to ensure care for the person.

MONITOR THE IMPACT OF ROLE RESTRUCTURING

Methods for assessing the impact of an intervention are critical to measuring success, so therapists need to monitor the effects of their efforts to shift family caregiving roles. Role restructuring typically is measured in terms of changes in actual behavior. Exactly what different care services are the caregivers providing? Exactly what behaviors are other family members doing to support the primary caregiver? How do the caregiver and care recipient interact differently?

The original data used to assess caregiver role structure issues can be used to track change in response to intervention. These include

- alignment between care recipient's care needs and the services provided by the overall caregiving structure;
- distribution of care tasks among the caregivers such that decision-making authority is clear, roles are well defined, and the primary caregiver feels supported;

- pathways of communication exist for renegotiating roles as the care recipient's or caregiver's needs change; and
- the primary caregiver's role identity is congruent with the caregiving roles needed by the care recipient.

Conclusion

Perhaps the most daunting task faced by caregivers of adults is changing the family roles in the ways needed to accomplish the work that must be done while supporting the ongoing development of all members. The current generation of older adults will receive care in contexts so different from previous generations' experiences that their caregivers have little personal history from which to draw guidance. Family structures can constrain or open possibilities for caregivers. Core structural characteristics or the dynamics that shape the way structures function within particular families all serve as the salient backdrop for caregiving activities within families. A common structure associated with successful caregiving is the identification of a primary caregiver along with secondary caregivers who play a support role to the primary caregiver as well as the care recipient. Key questions faced by families in organizing their caregiving structures include how various roles are valued and the identity of the caregiver role.

Families often need guidance to recognize the type of role transition needed and the contexts that make the transition challenging, as well as to find new ways of interacting that open doors for full role changes. Role changes are implemented as changes in behavior or verbal communication that reflect different positions within the family for care recipient and care provider. Therapists need to be clear about the values dimensions along which role transitions occur. Proactive intervention strategies help family members try out new role structures. Ongoing tracking of behavior changes in role implementation patterns assesses intervention success.

Role Reverberations 5

The transition into the role of caregiver for an older family member usually involves a steep learning curve. The role acquisition period, a time when the components of the new role are being learned, is quite demanding, as documented in an important study of dementia caregivers by Aneshensel, Pearlin, Mullan, Zarit, and Whitlatch (1995). This chapter outlines some of the challenges inherent in taking on a new role: learning the demands of the role, managing the strains that accompany the addition of a new role to the existing ones, and handling the interpersonal challenges with other family members that can arise (case descriptions of this stage elaborated in Chapter 8).

Assuming that the caregiving role has been shaped to be appropriate to the needs of the care recipient, the caregiver family therapy (CFT) therapist now turns attention to helping the caregiver implement the role within the context of existing roles, relationships, and other life demands. The CFT model will proceed from this point of reflection on the bigger picture of how caregiving fits within the caregiver's

DOI: 10.1037/13943-005
Caregiver Family Therapy: Empowering Families to Meet the Challenges of Aging,
by S. H. Qualls and A. A. Williams

overall life, toward a more focused consideration of caregiver self-care in the next three chapters. However, before self-care strategies can be developed, the therapist and the caregiver need a rich understanding of the costs of the caregiving role and its consequences for other life structures. That exploration begins with a thorough understanding of role demands.

Role Implementation Challenges

Previous steps in the CFT process engaged the therapist and the family in defining clearly the care demands and organizing the caregiving role(s) around the care recipient's needs as well as the caregiver's skills. A role structure was created within the family in which particular people were identified to engage in particular tasks to support their loved one. The therapist needs to watch carefully as the family implements this role structure. Two key questions now need to be monitored by the therapist and primary caregiver:

- Does each family member have the skills and knowledge needed to actually do the tasks they agreed to do?
- Are the role structures sustainable for each caregiver without risking burnout in the caregiver role or in other life roles (e.g., work, family)?

Caregiver's Knowledge and Skills

Like any other job or career, caregiving roles often include components that stretch the caregiver into new territory, well past known knowledge and skills (Aneshensel et al., 1995; McDaniel, 1995; McDaniel, Hepworth, & Doherty, 1992; Rolland, 1994). Family members may be expected to insert catheters, manage complicated medical regimens, and navigate complex health systems. Not surprisingly, caregivers do not know what they do not know when they take on the role, so they may be quite unprepared for the level of work involved during the role acquisition phase. Therapists need to check in on the impact of the role structure once it has been implemented because clients may be surprised by what they experience once the plan is set in motion.

FIGURE 5.1

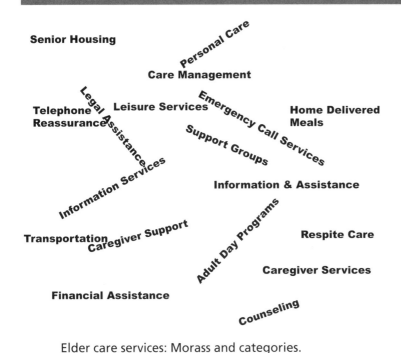

Senior Housing
- Independent
- Assisted Living
- Skilled Nursing

Senior Services
- Day Programs
- In–Home Care
- Transportation
- Meals
- Disease–support Organizations
- Care Management

Health Care
- Hospital
- Primary
- Specialty
- Mental Health

Senior Housing
Personal Care
Care Management
Telephone Reassurance
Legal Assistance
Leisure Services
Emergency Call Services
Home Delivered Meals
Support Groups
Information Services
Information & Assistance
Transportation
Caregiver Support
Adult Day Programs
Respite Care
Caregiver Services
Financial Assistance
Counseling

Elder care services: Morass and categories.

Therapists need to be sensitive to the learning curve on which caregivers find themselves and assist them in locating the resources needed. Obviously, therapists need to know this information, and those new to chronic disease work with older adults will have their own steep learning curve. Therapists simply must invest time and effort to build knowledge of care delivery systems (e.g., housing, health care, social services), funding streams for various services, legal and financial tools, and many other resources. Initially, therapists and families experience the services networks as if they were the morass of uncoordinated services depicted on the left side of Figure 5.1. Over time, the internal structure of the services network will become more evident.

CFT therapists can help orient families to the categories of resources (see the right side of Figure 5.1) and identify access points in the particular region in which the older family member lives. As described in Chapter 3 of this volume, points of entry to learn about services in the United States are almost always available through the Area Agency on Aging (AAA) network (http://www.eldercare.gov). Online access directs the seeker to the nearest AAA, where an information and assistance telephone line is staffed by persons ready to assist the family in locating services. Some AAAs also offer counseling services to caregivers, but all offer extraordinarily helpful service listings.

Caregivers provide a remarkable level of technical health care services as well, which usually is new to them. Family members may be in charge of changing a catheter, transferring someone from bed to chair, dispensing complex medication regimens, preparing and serving meals that meet very specific nutritional requirements, cleaning wounds, managing broken-down skin, organizing medical appointments, archiving medical information, and so on. Durable medical equipment and prosthetic devices are ubiquitous in geriatric health care. Oxygen tanks, bathing chairs, special stockings, wheelchairs, and walkers—all of which are routine aspects of daily life in home-based care—require skill to operate or support another in using.

Despite these responsibilities, family members are rarely included in the communication loop of the health care team. Family questions are practical ones that service systems are not always prepared to answer straightforwardly. As a single example, consider the family dilemma about whether it is time to take away driving privileges. This question probably requires that an answer be pieced together from a virtual team of professionals, including primary care provider and neuropsychologist, with input potentially from an occupational therapist, lawyer, neurologist, and psychiatrist, among others. The family holds onto the practical care question while engaging professionals one by one and figuring out how to get them to integrate their answers. The skills needed to manage this level of care coordination are substantial enough to command a meaningful salary for professionals in the health care field!

Ironically, the formal care plan that is orchestrated by the primary care physician is likely to have never been shared with the spouse who retains the 24/7 care responsibility. Furthermore, family members are often shocked to learn that the various providers all have separate care plans that have rarely been shared, let alone integrated into a single overarching plan. In short, families are part of a virtual team that is poorly or not coordinated, let alone integrated, and the family members are explicitly excluded from that team yet are presumed to offer 24/7 care with knowledge and skill. Despite the availability of sophisticated electronic technologies in all sectors of our society, simple communication among members of the team is not well scripted or supported.

Therapists can assist families during this stressful role acquisition phase with information, resources and referrals, and guidance in how to navigate systems. A single call to the AAA's information and assistance telephone line system in the region where the care recipient resides generates significant resource information, usually in the form of a list of providers of a desired service. Navigating the system, however, requires a more complex and nuanced knowledge and skill set that therapists become more capable of sharing as their own experience base grows.

For example, if a daughter wants to direct the physician's attention to a problem her mother is unlikely to mention, she can fax a letter or statement of concern to the physician or nurse. Therapists can help clients write a brief statement of concern with pertinent observation data that would not otherwise be available to the physician, including a specific action request. The written documentation almost always becomes a part of the patient's chart and thus is a leverage point for generating action. The daughter can also fax to the physician a signed statement of approval for the physician to discuss her mother's health care with her, opening the avenue of a telephone conversation in which the physician or nurse can share specific information from the evaluation that otherwise would be considered privileged health information. Similarly, specific hints can help families navigate assisted living staff structures that seem daunting to them otherwise.

Impact on Caregivers' Well-Being

CFT requires the therapist to revisit the role structures that are in place to deliver care with an eye to the impact on the caregiver's life and well-being. Some role structures that work well on paper simply cannot be sustained because the cost to the caregiver's well-being is too high. Other role structures are entirely possible if the family is provided with the information, training, and support to implement them successfully. Therapists work with the caregiver family to anticipate gaps in knowledge and training that can be filled before a crisis arises.

The therapist needs to lead the inquiry into the impact of caregiving on the caregiver because families simply cannot understand the scope or weight of responsibility they take on when attempting to provide care unless they have experience with this specific problem. Caregivers who provide care over an extended period show a suppressed immune response that makes them vulnerable to their own health problems (Kiecolt-Glaser, Dura, Speicher, Trask, & Glaser, 1991). Spouses whose advanced age makes them highly likely to have their own health challenges can easily become physically weary, at risk for illness or accident before those around them recognize the problem.

In sum, CFT therapists must follow any role renegotiation or restructuring with careful attention to empowering the caregiver to gain the knowledge and skills necessary to implement the role. The role acquisition phase is likely to be exhausting as the caregiver learns how to navigate complex systems of care that are poorly coordinated. The role's demands need to be monitored carefully to ensure that they are not overloading the caregiver beyond sustainability. Revisiting the role structure may be necessary before finalizing the structure for this phase of caregiving, with the option of investigating whether formal care partners need to be hired to support the role of the primary caregiver.

Key questions to ask the caregiver include the following (Anderson et al., 2008):

- When you wake up in the morning, what do you look forward to most? What do you look forward to least?
- What are the best things about being (e.g., a mother, a wife, an employee)? What are the most challenging things?
- Which caregiving tasks are easy for you, and which are hard?
- How do the rewards and challenges from one area in your life impact another area?

Role Structure Risks: Overloads, Traps, and Strains

OVERLOAD

Many caregivers are at risk for feeling overloaded—they simply have too many roles for any one person to perform without becoming exhausted. Caregivers who are providing a large number of activities of daily living (ADLs) and instrumental activities of daily living (IADLs) are likely to be overloaded, but even those handling far fewer tasks may feel overloaded if those tasks are unfamiliar, time consuming, or different from the past role patterns.

TRAPS

In addition to the potential for role overload, caregivers can end up feeling trapped in the role. Regardless of whether they embraced it initially, they may end up feeling that they carry a burden for which there is no escape. The feelings of being burdened and stressed have predicted poor outcomes for caregivers in multiple research studies (Knight & Losada, 2011; Pinquart & Sörensen, 2005a).

Choice is the route out of feeling trapped. Some caregivers can remind themselves that they have chosen this path, and that is sufficient to ward off the panic and despair of feeling trapped. Even if they have to remind themselves every day, essentially they can shift

EXHIBIT 5.1

Jack

When Sadie had a stroke, her husband, Jack, immediately took on the role of caregiver. He carefully followed her through the inpatient rehabilitation stay, taking copious notes on how to exercise her weakened left side. He also took over all household responsibilities for shopping, cooking, cleaning, coordinating communication with children, and gift purchasing for special events. When Sadie was discharged home, Jack added the following roles:

- physical therapist to retrain her to walk;
- occupational therapist to train her how to feed and assist with dressing herself;
- activity director to keep her entertained despite difficulty with attention and language;
- household manager to sanitize the frequently soiled sheets and clothing;
- nurse to manage catheter care, medication administration, and urine and bowel output monitoring;
- nurse's aide to respond to the call bell that rang about every 15 minutes, transferring her to bedside commode or wheelchair, and back to bed;
- transport service to get her in and out of the car and to myriad follow-up doctor appointments; and
- chaplain to address her existential despair over not regaining her life back fully.

The learning curve Jack faced was not just a short-term challenge. Not only did he have to acquire a wide array of skills, he also had to figure out how to sustain implementing them. In addition, Jack was living in a sleep-deprived stupor from Sadie's constant nighttime awakenings. He had his own health to manage as well. Somewhere in every 24 hours he also needed to communicate with family and friends about "how it was going." He was too tired to even consider the value of hiring help and ignorant of how he might do that if he wanted to do so.

After several months of observing him provide this extraordinary level of care, Jack's children confronted him with his obvious level of exhaustion. They insisted that he either accept in-home paid help or arrange to place Sadie into a residential facility. Jack acknowledged that he was exhausted but insisted that caring for Sadie at home was what he wanted to do as long as possible. The children convinced him to hire help that would allow him to exercise, attend his long-term service club meeting, church, and one lunch outing each week.

A few months later, the family checked back in and found that Jack showed less obvious strain on his face and generally appeared more relaxed. Although he reported that working with the paid home-care staff was harder than coordinating her care alone, he also acknowledged that he enjoyed being free to socialize and exercise, even limitedly. The children observed that he also exhibited more patience in his interactions with Sadie.

their focus so that they feel free to give rather than trapped by the role. Other caregivers need choices that remove or shift the workload. Sharing the caregiving tasks with other people is one pathway out of a trap. Secondary caregivers within the family may step up to do more of the work or to provide a break for a few hours, a day, or a week. Other caregivers determine that partnering with formal providers who are paid to do work on a predictable schedule provides the most relief (see the example in Exhibit 5.1). The social services industry refers to brief breaks (hours or days) for the caregiver as *respite care.*

STRAINS

Strain can refer to strain experienced in doing the tasks of a given role or to strain experienced because of competing demands among roles. A wife and mother of teenagers whose 8-to-5 job is demanding really has little emotional energy or time to take on oversight or care of a frail older adult who needs close supervision. Inevitably, any caregiver role she adopts for the older family member will require her to change some aspects of her other roles.

Research on caregiver strain yields a more complex picture than the simple notion that more roles lead to more role strain, however. Certainly, more roles can create a sense of being flooded by one more set of demands. A caregiver may turn to the role of caring for the older adult as a joyful respite from the challenges of rearing teenagers or a boring or difficult job. Indeed, caregivers report more rewards than stresses and in some circumstances report that the care they provide for an older family member helps sustain them in their other roles. Furthermore, paid employment does not necessarily add role burden, because highly rewarding work can be viewed as enhancing the caregiving role (Stephens & Franks, 2009). The bottom line is that in structuring caregiving roles, therapists need to be sensitive to both possibilities and assess each individual situation carefully.

Key questions to consider include the following:

- How does your new role impact roles you once had (e.g., being a mother, a wife, an employee, a friend)?
- How does your role impact your other current roles (e.g., are you not attending to other roles because caregiving is all consuming)?

Competing Role Demands

Any family genogram shows structural information about family roles (e.g., parenting, sibling connections, spouse/partner), but further investigation is needed to understand the meaning of those roles. For example, are there family members who require unusual care and oversight? Who is experiencing heavy responsibility for child rearing? Has divorce perhaps disbursed parenting roles among grandparents or others whose support supplements the primary parents' roles? Are ex-spouses still involved in caring for members of the family with whom they have had decades of experience?

Figure 5.2 shows an example of a simple pie chart task that can help caregivers sort out the amount of investment needed in various roles. A

FIGURE 5.2

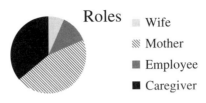

Role map.

therapist can help a caregiver reflect on role challenges by encouraging him or her to generate a list of roles and draw a pie chart that illustrates the amount of time spent in each. As needed, the therapist might direct the client to draw another chart to depict the way the client would like his or her time to be allocated among those roles, or the caregiver might need to draw a pie chart depicting the value or importance of each role to compare with the time spent in the role (Anderson et al., 2008; Ducharme et al., 2003).

The primary caregiver's competing role demands need to be reviewed in light of the current caregiving role responsibilities. What does the caregiver client need to do, and choose to do, for family members other than the older adult care recipient? What resources are available to assist with any of those demands (e.g., babysitters for small children, funding for college expenses, housecleaning services, in-home respite care)? Even relationships that are not explicitly identified with caregiving require care and feeding in order to be healthy. What types of nurturance are invested in the caregiver's marriage, sibling relationships, or adult children and grandchildren? The therapist needs to track the level of emotional demands as well as time-and-effort demands that are offered or extracted in the array of relationships in which the caregiver is embedded.

Nonfamilial roles need to be investigated as well. Many roles exist outside the family, such as worker, community leader, or religious institution leader. Information from a typical intake form will suggest roles that need to be investigated. Key questions include the amount of time commitment involved in the roles, the level of responsibility, whether they require steady or intermittent involvement, and the current level of stress associated with each. Family caregivers of aging people also have other dimensions to their lives that influence directly and indirectly their capability to carry out various caregiving tasks and roles.

Key questions to ask the caregiver include the following:

- What roles do you currently play in your life?
- What activities did you used to do but had to give up when you began caregiving?

- What impacts how much time you allocate to each role?
- How do you account for the differences between your present and desired role-time allocations?
- What do you wish you had more time for?

Competing demands cannot be assumed to be inherently positive or negative (Stephens & Franks, 2009). Nor are they even static in their impact on individuals; some roles cycle in their demands or their emotional impact on individuals. The strategies used to adapt to multiple role demands are also key to investigate because they determine whether caregiving will compete with, complement, or enhance other roles. Some caregivers describe the quiet time they spend in a parent's nursing home room as the only silent down time of their day, a welcome respite between work and child-rearing demands. Stopping by the nursing home daily may be a very positive benefit to them, as opposed to a drain. Others, however, have given up exercise to make the same daily visit to a family member in a facility. The meaning of each role and role-related task, along with the structural characteristics of the role that might influence caregiving (e.g., time, static/intermittent role loads, stress), need to be explored in an interview to complete understanding of the implicit as well as explicit demands of various roles.

Of course, these potential role strains from competing demands are not relevant solely to the primary caregiver but also apply to secondary caregivers. Siblings may agree to take turns visiting parents who live at a distance as support for the primary spousal caregiver. The same monthly or quarterly rotation is unlikely to have the same impact on the siblings. For example, one sibling has school-age children and must hire a sitter to oversee them for the weekend when she is with the parents. Another sibling may have financial challenges that make the cost of a cross-country flight a significant burden. Yet another may travel with a spouse so they can provide double the level of care support while visiting. The effects of care roles on competing role demands need to be examined for all members of the family to ensure that the chosen role structure at least appears to be truly sustainable over time.

Families also need to be given permission to review the structure regularly with an eye to making changes as needed. Recalibration of role structures should be expected so that family structures do not ossify. Many factors will require readjustment of structures over time, including misjudgment of the role structures that are needed, changes in care recipient needs, inability to sustain over time what appeared to be viable initially, changes in caregivers' lives, and changes in resource availability. Therapists will find it useful to name the current structure as the best guess for today as to what is needed and useful, with the clear understanding that recalibration is very likely to be needed.

Regular Role Checkups

Anticipating the need to adjust roles, the therapist can help the family prepare a strategy for reviewing role assignments and requesting revisions. An established date for a formal review takes the burden off of the caregivers to be the one(s) to ask the family for help. A semi-annual review might be assigned to someone in the family to initiate. Perhaps the person who attends the health visits with the care recipient is assigned to report back to other family members and tasked with raising questions at that point about how everyone is coping with the current structure. The family might want to set an appointment with the therapist as a commitment to conduct the review and to ensure that someone can facilitate a thorough conversation. Formal providers may use care conferences that add information to the family's assessment. Rarely do care conferences do a thorough review of the family care structures, however, so families should not expect assistance with reviewing their role structures from care conferences.

Key questions to include in that caregiver role check-in might be:

- What does the health provider see as changing? Any revision in health treatment plans?
- Does anyone in the family see changes in the care recipient's ability to do ADLs and IADLs? How have those been accommodated so far?
- How is the primary caregiver doing physically? emotionally? socially?
- How is the division of responsibility among family members working out? What challenges (we often call them "rubs") have arisen? Are any substantial enough to require a full role structure discussion?
- Has anyone learned information about external resources that he or she would like to share with the rest of the family?

Interpersonal Role Challenges

Caregiving role structures that work quite effectively for the primary caregiver and the care recipient can ruffle feathers among other family members who dislike the role configuration, disagree with what is to be done, or experience negative effects secondary to the caregiving role structures. Some of the most challenging CFT work occurs when the family members are in conflict among themselves as to how they should provide care or live with the consequences of caregiving. Often, the war is framed as a moral one, with battle lines drawn around care strategies as if they reflect good and bad ways of being a family.

Chronic diseases plop a very significant level of challenge in the middle of the ongoing complexities of family development (McDaniel, 1995). All normal developmental transitions challenge families, and some families simply struggle with almost every transition that engages the family in role changes. Change comes hard in families that are highly rigid in their rules and roles, as well as in those who are so chaotic they lack patterns to use in adapting. More flexible families still face significant adjustment when caregiving demands are positioned within the ongoing activities of a normal family.

Even if family members agree with who should be the caregiver, they may disagree with what is to be done, so new conflicts can arise after a caregiving structure has been put into place. Caregivers' choices about how to provide care are often viewed by others as unnecessary, overbearing, inappropriate, inadequate, or inconsistent with the care recipient's previously stated preferences. Such differences of opinion about care may be stated in language far more emotionally loaded than a simple statement of care preference:

- "You just don't care what Mom wanted, it's all about you."
- "Since when does Dad's money flow freely to you for caring for him when our sister took care of him for years for free?"
- "You know that you wouldn't care one whit about whether he goes to church, but you don't want the pastor snooping around into his affairs."

Interpersonal conflicts that arise as care strategies and care structures are implemented can be highly disruptive to both the primary caregiver and the care recipient. A major benefit to families of using CFT is that they can anticipate some of the challenges before they arise, so that fewer people are surprised by how the care plan really works (and does not). Obviously, the therapist plays a significant role in this normalizing procedure, inviting the family to picture challenges that may arise even before the plan is implemented. The family member client also can be invited to think through who else needs to be educated about those potential challenges before they arise. As they begin to discharge their new roles, caregivers will likely have little buffer space available to handle others' upset feelings.

Family members who were not on the client's radar screen during the initial work now may have highly salient reactions to the care plan as it is implemented. Even if inoculated to the potential for new conflicts to arise, caregivers are likely to feel ambushed or undermined by other family members who now voice strong opinions about or reactions to the care plan. For example:

- "That place is awful—we cannot begin to think about leaving Dad there. What were you thinking?"
- "Why in the world did you let them take her keys away when there is not one piece of evidence that her driving is a problem?"
- "You should never have let them transfer her to the hospital—good things never happen in hospitals."
- "She needs a haircut and style. Why do you let her look so awful?"
- "You just let that doctor talk you into trying an experimental medication without thinking about what bad things could happen! You need to be more careful."

Family members who are surprised or shocked by seeing how the care system really works can easily lash out at the person who set up the plan, without thinking that he or she is just as distressed by what is happening.

Older adults worry about conflicts within their families, and families often find it difficult to keep conflict a secret from a care recipient. This fact is a piece of leverage for the therapist to use in calling the family to work toward resolution. Families are sometimes directed to CFT because the care recipient is distressed about the conflict within the family. Formal care providers such as housing administrators or health care providers may become caught in the middle of feuding families and realize that the conflict is disrupting care delivery. When formal providers are care partners, they also may be able to provide an independent assessment of the level of disruption experienced by the care recipient. The CFT therapist may request an independent interview with the care recipient or may ask another provider to gather information about the care recipient's reaction to the conflict within the family. If the care recipient is in fact distressed about the conflict, individual psychotherapy or counseling should be made available to the older adult to help him or her work through the nearly inevitable guilt about "being such a burden to the children that they are fighting about me." The older adult may also be invited into a therapy session with other family members to help the feuding parties recognize the negative effects of their conflict on the very person they are attempting to help.

The process of calling family members to work together usually requires the therapist to walk the family back through the previous steps in CFT (naming, care structuring, role structuring). A deliberate review of that process may seem time consuming, but it is very important to give all members a chance to work through resistance to the problem itself, the constraints within the family (e.g., resources) for solving the problem, and the options for structuring care and caregiving roles.

Many strategies can be used to invite the family together, so therapist and caregiver client need to work together to identify an optimal strategy for that family. A timed check can be referenced as if it were an objective, externally generated reason to meet. "We are approaching the 3-month point, so we need to sit down together to review what has happened since we started ____ ." Similarly, the family may rely on an external person to signal them when it is time to meet. "John's case worker says we need to review the care plan because quite a bit has changed recently and we need to think about how to modify the plan accordingly." The client can make a personal plea for her or his own benefit. For example:

- "I would really appreciate if you would attend a meeting with my caregiving coach/counselor/therapist to give me input where she can help me hear all of what concerns you."
- "As you know, I have been serving as the primary overseer of Mother's care since last summer, and I would really appreciate your observations and insights into the care she is getting at the assisted living facility."
- "I'm starting to worry that the current plan is not going to last forever so would really appreciate the chance to brainstorm with you the next set of options."

Finally, a family member can refer directly to the conflict or feud as an important reason to meet. For example:

- "I know that you have not agreed with my choices about your father's care, and I recognize that I have not really asked why before, but I am now ready to hear your input even if it is not going to be easy."
- "I hear from others in the family that you are pretty angry with me for ____ , and I'll admit that scares me a bit, but I really would like to get to the bottom of this before the holidays so we can be together with mom/dad/sister without any big fight because I realize he/she doesn't need that."

Although we are expert at reacting intensely within our families, we often do not know how to build a bridge over the troubled waters. CFT therapists need to be prepared to help family caregivers navigate what seems almost inevitable, conflict over implementation of care structures and strategies. Conflict is easier to handle if someone helped the family anticipate the fact that the journey is not going to be smooth and that all care plans are an experiment that can be revised and revisited over time.

Family caregivers are truly challenged to hear disagreements over care plans and strategies without taking the input personally. Often the statement of disagreement is a messy, mixed message delivered with emotional intensity bubbling up from under the surface. Even the most centered, emotionally healthy, wise person will be hard pressed to walk for months or years along the rollercoaster journey that is chronic disease management and care without finding some pretty major potholes in the road. The primary caregiver is perhaps the most vulnerable person, next to the care recipient himself or herself. CFT therapists seek ways to review regularly the impact of care structures and strategies as they are implemented over time.

Conclusion

This step between two of the core processes in the CFT model is intended to offer the therapist and primary caregiver a moment in which to review the viability of the roles structures that were renegotiated. This review process examines the viability of the roles and strategies to meet the objective role demands; avoid subjective distress from role overload, strain, or entrapment; and proactively address interpersonal conflicts that might arise from the ways in which roles are structured. Caregivers will not implement critical self-care strategies if they do not see the roles as viable. Therapists are wise to do a careful review of the long-term sustainability of the new role structures as well as the interpersonal implications of those structures before attempting to engage the caregiver in self-care efforts.

Caregiver Self-Care 6

S elf-care, as a concept, is applied very broadly in the caregiver family therapy (CFT) program to individual well-being in the context of the family system. Consistent with other multi-dimensional models of intervention (e.g., Mittelman, Roth, Clay, & Haley, 2007), CFT focuses on the whole person in multiple domains of life and adds a focus on the family system as a salient context for caregiver functioning and well-being.

Information about the caregiver's well-being may have shaped the choices of problems to address in earlier phases of CFT but likely did not become the central focus of the earliest sessions of CFT unless the caregiver was at immediate risk of deleterious outcomes without crisis intervention. Instead, the early focus is more commonly on naming the problem and then problem solving to meet care recipients' needs first. Role reconfiguration is often needed just to meet care recipients' needs and again certainly includes conscious attention to caregivers' well-being as a factor in the choice of how to configure roles. The current step in CFT, however, focuses

DOI: 10.1037/13943-006
Caregiver Family Therapy: Empowering Families to Meet the Challenges of Aging,
by S. H. Qualls and A. A. Williams

in a deep, rich way on caregiver self-care to sustain whatever approaches were selected to meet the care recipient's ongoing care needs. This chapter outlines a rationale for caregivers to invest in self-care, applies the biopsychosocial model of care to caregiver well-being, and suggests strategies for bypassing caregivers' resistance to self-care (case descriptions of this stage provided in Chapter 8).

Importance of Self-Care to Well-Being

Caregiving has negative effects on long-term health and well-being (Schultz & Martire, 2004; Vitaliano, Young, & Zhang, 2004) and immune function (Kiecolt-Glaser et al., 1987) and is associated with high rates of mortality and morbidity (Schulz, 1995; Schulz & Beach, 1999). What are the causes of these deleterious health effects of caregiving? Older adults have more chronic illnesses than younger and middle-age adults, and caregiving adds increased risk for physical illnesses above and beyond the risks associated with typical aging (Liu & Gallagher-Thompson, 2009; Pinquart & Sorensen, 2007). Caregivers are vulnerable to acute and chronic illnesses in part because of compromised immune function following extended periods of caregiving and in part because of age-related risk factors that are likely present, in spousal caregivers in particular (Cacioppo et al., 1998; Kiecolt-Glaser et al., 1991).

Caregiving is a long-term stressor, and those caregivers who always engaged in sufficient self-care activities need to make extraordinary efforts to continue doing so or experience risk to their health (Zarit, Orr, & Zarit, 1985). Yet caregivers, compared with noncaregivers, encounter more barriers to self-care, have lower self-efficacy related to self-care behaviors, engage in less physical activity, and get fewer hours of sleep (Acton, 2002). Caregivers also rate "health responsibility, spiritual growth, interpersonal relationships, and stress management" lower than do noncaregivers (Acton, 2002, p. 81). Acton's (2002) findings suggest that caregivers who engage in more health-promoting activities experience less stress and better overall well-being than those caregivers who engage in few such self-care activities.

All spiritual, mental health, and physical health paradigms recognize the importance of self-care. Self-care is a shared value in the American culture despite society's failure to promote it very well. Competing demands are almost always at play, and individuals find themselves struggling to make it to the gym when they have a deadline at work or when adolescent sons or daughters have their own after-school activities. CFT therapists work with caregivers to bring self-care activities to the forefront in terms of setting priorities because caregivers who engage in self-care have better overall well-being and are therefore able to provide care more adequately to their care recipients.

Many caregivers come into therapy with an awareness that self-care is important, if not essential, to the caregiving process. However, in the majority of cases, caregivers find it difficult to implement suggestions revolving around self-care because they tend to put others' needs ahead of their own. Teaching a caregiver that his or her self-care is linked to care recipient well-being helps the caregiver make taking care of himself or herself more of a priority. For example, a caregiver who is spread too thin may become drained or ill and then be unable, at least temporarily, to attend to the care recipient. An overwhelmed caregiver may also be more likely to have an accident and sustain an injury, which could keep him or her from being able to provide adequate care.

Components of Self-Care

Self-care, by definition, involves caregivers acknowledging and attending to their own physical, psychological, and social needs. This requires them, first and foremost, to understand that each person is responsible for managing his or her own well-being while at the same time attending to the needs of another person. Self-care includes a range of pleasurable activities, such as reading and visiting with friends, and health-promoting actions, such as adequate sleep and appropriate exercise (Acton, 2002, p. 73). These activities help to reduce stress and maintain a sense of balance in life, thus improving the caregiver's quality of life both physically and emotionally. Several factors associated with self-care activities (i.e., social support, physical health, quality of relationships) may moderate the progressive negative effects of caregiving, such as burnout and poor health outcomes (Sörensen & Conwell, 2011). Caregiver burnout occurs when an individual feels overwhelmed, under duress, and consequently as if they cannot carry on their current caregiving load while balancing it with life outside of caregiving (Figley, 1998).

Role of CFT in Promoting Self-Care

The overall goals in the self-care phase of CFT are to assist caregivers in identifying and assessing stressors and self-care activities, learning goal-setting techniques to initiate these self-care activities, sustaining the activities, evaluating stress levels and activity effectiveness, and thus managing caregiver burden and associated stressors (Coon, Gallagher-Thompson, & Thompson, 2003). Further objectives of this phase of therapy are to improve the caregiver's quality of life as he or she learns to increase effective care and to decrease possible resentment toward the care recipient or other family members whose involvement in caregiving is a point of concern. Specifically, self-care involves the caregiver attending to his or her own physical, psychological, and sociocultural needs during the caregiving journey (S. H. Jones, 2007).

CFT therapists must also talk with caregivers about preparing for times when they could suddenly be unable to provide care to the recipient. If the caregiver has not taken steps to prepare for alternate caregivers to step in and help, the care recipient will be at risk while such arrangements are being made. Unfortunately, the majority of caregivers do not plan, perhaps because they believe that no one else can step in and provide the same level of care or perhaps because of simple denial of risk to self. The CFT therapist will want to assess caregivers' beliefs about preparing for worst-case scenarios as well as how they feel about taking time for themselves.

Caregivers are diverse in terms of their needs when they enter CFT, and these can change over time. For example, even if a caregiver is healthy physically and psychologically and has an active social life upon entering CFT, his or her psychological well-being may deteriorate as the caregiving journey continues (see the example in Exhibit 6.1). He or she may develop poor sleep and appetite patterns, worry about managing caregiving, experience strain from thinking about other family members' health and well-being, cease participating in social activities, and develop any number of other symptoms. Thus, the CFT therapist should assess the caregiver's self-care needs at varying points in the caregiving journey.

Effect of Care Recipient Functioning on Caregiver Self-Care Goals

Care recipient functioning also influences the caregiver's self-care goals and strategies for reaching them. The caregiver's self-care activities must correspond with the needs of the care recipient in ways that do not leave the latter vulnerable to harm or neglect. For example, a caregiver who struggles with a personality disorder or a mood disorder may at times be less focused on the care recipient than necessary,

Mr. Wright

Mr. Wright is a caregiver for his father and mother, who live together about 5 miles away from Mr. Wright. Mr. Wright lives with his wife and 20-year-old daughter, who goes to the community college nearby. Mr. Wright has been caring for his father, who has Alzheimer's disease, and his mother, who has osteoporosis but is otherwise healthy, for the past 3 years. He drives his parents to their appointments, fixes things around their house, and assists his mother with day-to-day tasks related to caring for his father. In addition to caregiving, Mr. Wright works full time as a manager at a small family-owned hardware store. He loves his job and finds it rewarding to talk with customers and teach employees about home-modification projects and tools. Mr. Wright and his wife make it a point to spend time together every weekend, either doing a project around their own home, gardening, or taking a trip into the mountains for a day of rest and relaxation. The Wrights decided together that they wanted to ask their daughter to continue to live at home while she attends college to support her financially until she graduates and finds a job. Mr. Wright describes his relationship with his daughter as "close," and he tells his therapist that she has always been a source of pride for him. Mr. Wright also has a son who lives about an hour away and with whom he has a somewhat contentious relationship. Mr. Wright explains that he and his son are "too much alike to see eye-to-eye much of the time." In addition to work and family commitments, Mr. Wright indicates that he has friends with whom he spends time once in awhile, he attends church weekly, and he likes going fishing, although he has recently found that he has less time available for outdoor recreation than in the past.

After 6 months of therapy, Mr. Wright reports that his wife will begin treatment for cancer, all at the same time that Mr. Wright is caring for his parents and supporting his daughter. Mr. Wright's therapist, as she talks with him about self-care, must take into consideration the complexity of the family's current situation, including both the caregiver's and care recipient's functioning. The therapist's guidance at this point in his caregiving journey is much more focused on self-care than when Mr. Wright first came in for therapy, before his wife also became ill.

blaming latter for his or her problems instead of realizing that the care recipient legitimately needs support. In such a case, the CFT therapist will want to emphasize self-care activities for the caregiver that pay particular attention to the needs of the care recipient. If a break from caregiving is recommended, then the CFT therapist will want to counsel the caregiver to make sure that adequate respite providers are in place. In other cases, very well-intentioned caregivers may make plans for a family trip that includes the care recipient without thinking through all of the care recipient's needs. An overseas flight, stays in hotels, and lengthy day trips that include a great deal of walking may not be realistic for a care recipient who has had a stroke or uses an oxygen supply, for example. CFT therapists can help caregivers think through the details of upcoming events that are focused on self-care to make sure that both their own and the care recipient's needs will be met.

Caregiving Challenges
Self-Care

Self-care activities can seem counterintuitive to caregivers when they are more accustomed to caring for others. The CFT therapist's job is to break through caregivers' practical and conceptual barriers to engaging in self-care activities. In some cases, caregivers may believe that they do not have any time available for self-care, and in many cases, they may be correct to an extent, yet they also cannot afford not to care for themselves.

Caregiving takes time from self-care. On average, caregivers spend 20.4 hours per week engaged in caregiving activities (National Alliance for Caregiving, 2009), so CFT therapists need to find out from individual caregivers exactly how their time is impacted by their caregiving responsibilities. In some cases, caregivers may not have initially had good self-care patterns and now likely experience extraordinary stress. CFT may be a caregiver's first opportunity to think carefully about self-care as the straw has now broken (or is about to break) the camel's back. Self-care in the caregiving context may look different from how it did in the past and may push caregivers to negotiate time explicitly for themselves, which is loaded with meaning for many. Exceptional self-care requires balancing self-care, caregiving for the older person, and other responsibilities (e.g., work, family).

When caregivers provide information about the most salient problems in their caregiving situations, they trigger personalized interventions in the self-care phase of CFT, just as they did in the problem-solving phase. For example, if a caregiver indicates that he or she is in trouble at work because of taking time off frequently to assist the care recipient, the therapist will want to assess many aspects of the caregiver's life to determine what is causing the absences and how loss of a job might compromise his or her finances and career goals. If a caregiver views the greatest problems as feelings of loss and grief, the therapist will likely focus an intervention on normalizing the situation with empathy, offering psychoeducation about stages of illness progression and recommending increased relaxation and pleasant events to counteract the sadness felt about the care recipient's decline in functioning.

Biopsychosocial Model for
Self-Care

Many components of the caregiver's functioning need to be explored in order to understand the caregiver's problems and their contexts. Within the biopsychosocial model, self-care involves physical, psychological, and social well-being. Physical well-being consists of both health-promoting activities and disease management. Psychological well-being entails addressing stress and burden associated with caregiving, increasing coping skills, and managing symptoms of preexisting mental health conditions when they are present. Finally, an awareness of the caregiver's social functioning allows the CFT therapist to tailor self-care interventions to fit each individual's circumstances. In these domains of functioning, teaching assertiveness, improving communication skills, and encouraging caregivers to ask for and accept help are core elements of self-care.

PHYSICAL SELF-CARE

Beginning with the biological factors in the biopsychosocial model, CFT therapists assess multiple domains of caregivers' physical well-being. Interventions are designed to enhance wellness as well as to address any health concerns or conditions. CFT therapists will assess caregivers' attention to regular health checkups, diet, nutrition, exercise, medication management, and sleep, as well as the physical demands of providing care.

Key questions to consider include the following:

- Have you noticed changes (e.g., in appetite, sleep patterns, finances, interests, social activities/life, intimacy, relationships with others) in your everyday life?
- Have you seen your primary care provider in the past year for a physical?
- Did your primary care provider recommend any tests or treatments for chronic illnesses?
- Are you regularly ill? What are your primary care provider's recommendations? Are you routinely following your provider's instructions?

Overall physical health needs to be evaluated by appropriate professionals, so CFT therapists cannot rely simply on the client's self-assessment. Therapists want to address caregivers' physical status by ensuring that illnesses are appropriately treated, medications are up to date and being administered appropriately, and functional abilities are maximized. They need to gather information about chronic conditions and changes in the frequency, intensity, or trajectory of acute illnesses or acute episodes within chronic conditions.

CFT therapists assess whether caregivers regularly attend health care checkups and whether specialists are needed and used appropriately. In some cases, the caregiver will not have been to see a primary care physician recently, and the therapist can encourage him or her to do so and report back about his or her physical health. If a caregiver is hesitant to take time to go to a doctor's appointment, the therapist may want to educate him or her about chronic health conditions associated with aging (as well as the effects of stress on physical well-being) while also noting that health problems that go undetected for long periods of time are likely to be more severe and more difficult to correct once they are detected. Weight gain, for example, results from poor health management and can lead to multiple physical illnesses, which can be difficult to reverse. Resistance to self-care behaviors is always important to understand and address directly using strategies described next.

Caregivers from lower socioeconomic statuses and from oppressed groups receive lower quality medical care, and some neglect their personal medical care because their access to medical providers is limited (S. H. Jones, 2007). The following external and internal needs and assets can be points of intervention for therapists as they focus on self-care (S. H. Jones, 2007):

- External physical needs:
    - transportation to medical appointments
    - medications
    - access to primary care physicians and specialists
    - medical equipment
- External physical assets:
    - community resources
    - cultural supports for physical wellness
- Internal needs:
    - attention to signs of physical distress
    - adjustment of behavior to address physical needs (resting when feeling worn down)
- Internal assets:
    - perceptions of the importance of physical health
    - attitudes about health-promoting activities

Attending to the external and internal needs and assets of caregivers can boost their self-care in all areas of their lives. Self-care interventions aimed at promoting physical well-being include having an awareness of physical illnesses, knowing about methods of addressing those illnesses, and attending to health promotion and stress reduction activities.

Several ways that caregivers can engage in health-promoting activities include eating healthy foods, exercising, and sleeping well at night (Acton, 2002). Additionally, CFT therapists want to know whether caregivers are managing the physical demands of providing care. Some caregivers develop back problems, for example, when they are attending to transferring a care recipient from the bed to a chair or pushing a heavy wheelchair.

PSYCHOLOGICAL SELF-CARE

CFT therapists assess and make recommendations related to psychological functioning within the biopsychosocial approach to CFT therapy. Caregiving involves stresses, strains, and opportunities, all of which affect risk factors for physical and mental health problems. Among the strongest predictors of mental health problems are a subjective sense of burden from providing care and the feeling of being trapped (Aneshensel, Pearlin, Mullan, Zarit, & Whitlatch, 1995; Zarit, Reever, & Bach-Peterson, 1980). Subjective sense of burden includes stress, tension, and anxiety related to caregiving (Lai, 2010). Caregivers who lack a sense of choice about their roles experience role entrapment (Gaugler et al., 2005), which is associated with poor outcomes. Occupational, financial, and relationship strains secondary to caregiving also increase the burdens of caregiving. Of equal importance are positive responses to caregiving, including meaning, purpose, and gratification for providing a loving service to another. Some caregivers describe how they have gained role competence as a caregiver that has enhanced their identity and self-esteem. Some caregivers provide serial care to people in their families as well as friends and neighbors. These caregivers often appear to define their self-worth in terms of whether they are providing care to someone, and they may continue in their caregiving roles until they are exhausted.

Assessment of psychological effects of caregiving begins with asking the caregiver to describe how he or she is feeling about the caregiving process and whether support has been forthcoming from other family members. Questionnaires and interview questions can assist the therapist here.

Key questions to consider include the following:

- How would you describe your caregiving experience?
- Do you often feel overwhelmed? Does that occur much of the time or specifically with caregiving activities?
- Do you feel you can continue the current load of caregiving activities?
- Are there times you wish you were no longer a caregiver? Describe these times. What was going on? How were you feeling?
- When you are distressed, how does this affect your ability to care for your care recipient?
- Do you have any mental health concerns, such as depression and/ or anxiety?
- How do you usually handle feelings of sadness and worry?
- Are you regularly experiencing stress, distress, and burden?
- How do you manage these emotions?

To assess psychological self-care, the therapist can ask questions about the caregiver's daily activities, including opportunities for nurturing his or her emotional, spiritual, and intellectual needs. Screening tools for depression, loneliness, anxiety, and other distress states can provide indicators of domains where the caregiver is having difficulty.

These questions not only help the CFT therapist to assess the caregiver's current self-care status but also allow the therapist to determine whether the caregiver has attended to self-care activities in the past. Caregivers who endorse that they are healthy and happy and that they have friends with whom they spend time may already have an understanding of the importance of self-care.

Assess Caregiver-Specific Stress: Burden, Role Entrapment, Resentment, and Anxiety

Screening tools and questionnaires can be very useful in many settings. Some therapists use depression or loneliness screening tools, along with burden or distress measures. Useful caregiver distress measures include the Zarit Burden Inventory (Zarit, Orr, & Zarit, 1985; Zarit, Reever, & Bach-Peterson, 1980); the Caregiver Strain Index (Robinson, 1983); and, for a broad range of mental health problems, the Brief Symptom Inventory (Derogatis & Melisaratos, 1983).

Our University of Colorado (CU) Aging Center team developed its own version, and other clinicians may wish to follow suit if existing measures do not tap specific issues related to the caregiver populations served. Our Caregiver Reaction Scale (Appendix A) was adapted from Pearlin, Mullan, Semple, and Skaff (1990) specifically to assist caregivers in giving details about their caregiving experiences and the types of difficulties that they are facing as a result of their caregiving situation in an efficient format. The measure contains eight subscales that assess a variety of components, including level of stress; loss; self-efficacy; coping mechanisms; family disagreements about caregiving; and secondary effects of caregiving on work, finances, and family. Preliminary psychometric studies have shown that the subscales have good internal validity (Anderson, 2011); additional reliability and validity research is in progress.

The goal of any of these measures is to elicit reports of caregiver well-being in varied domains of life that are known to affect caregiving so additional assessment can guide the therapy process quickly toward areas of greatest concern. Scales allow the therapist to assess intensity as well as content of concerns, contributing to the therapist's sense of whether the caregiver will be able to continue providing care as he or she has been and whether changes in the caregiving situation are needed now or in the near future. Regardless of the data gathering strategy, the CFT therapist must glean a sense of the primary stressors that each caregiver experiences.

The therapist also examines types and frequency of pleasurable activities as a basis for selecting and tracking therapeutic interventions designed to increase mood through pleasant event interventions.

Again, the information can be gleaned in interview or through a data gathering form such as the Caregiver Activities and Assistance form (Figure 6.1) that generates an estimate of how many hours per week a client spends completing caregiving activities. After the intake session, the CFT therapist monitors mental health functioning and caregiver stress on an ongoing basis, either by repeated administration of questionnaires or by asking clients specific questions about their well-being. New problems with stress, burden, depression, and anxiety can become apparent to the therapist throughout the course of therapy when caregivers relate their feelings about their caregiving situations. CFT therapists can track improvement in self-care on the basis of the caregiver's ability to enact new self-care routines and decreases in caregivers' stress levels, especially when associated with new challenges presented by the caregiving journey.

Assess Precaregiving Mental Health

In many cases, the therapist will find that caregivers experience depression, anxiety, burden, and distress related to their roles. In addition to these typical emotional reactions to caregiving situations, caregivers

FIGURE 6.1

CAREGIVER ACTIVITIES AND ASSISTANCE
Estimate number of hours engaged in caregiving activities:
____Hours spent doing laundry per week
____Hours planning/cooking meals per week
____Hours spent grocery shopping per week
____Hours of dust/vacuuming per week
____Hours cleaning bathrooms per week
____Hours cleaning care recipient area per week
____Hours cleaning kitchen, scrubbing floors per week
____Hours spent supervising care recipient per week
____Hours bathing and hygiene care of recipient per week
____Hours of home maintenance for care recipient per week (yard work, home repairs, etc.)
____Hours of errands per week (picking up medications, shopping for hygiene products, etc.)
____Hours of banking/paying bills per week
____Hours driving to/attending appointments per month
____Hours communicating with relatives about care recipient's health and well-being
____Hours spent engaging in long-term care planning for care recipient
____Hours spent in other activities related to caregiving (providing medication to care recipient, etc.)
____Hours of self-care per week (time off from caregiver responsibilities, relaxation time,
     socialization, etc.)

Other activities of caregiving: taking care of immediate family needs, engaging in social activities, occupation…

Identify the current balance of time spent in caregiver activities versus self-care. What can be done to shift the balance?
What makes it difficult to maintain the balance?

Consider how others could be of help in certain areas. Reflect on what makes it difficult to ask others for help.

Caregiver activities and assistance form.

may also exhibit symptoms of long-standing mental health diagnoses, such as mood and personality disorders. Grief is also frequently a primary target for intervention in caregiver therapy, both during the caregiving process and after the care recipient dies. Furthermore, caregivers frequently experience conflict, guilt, irritability, and anger (S. H. Jones, 2007, p. 107). Clinicians, as they assess these areas of functioning, will be able to determine whether their caregiver clients are integrating self-care techniques into their day-to-day routines.

Assess Mood Management During Caregiving

CFT therapists are interested in how caregiving affects mood management, so they assess caregivers' engagement in pleasant events and ability to relax sufficiently to experience pleasure in them (Coon et al, 2003). CFT therapists may teach relaxation to caregivers who cannot focus on pleasure or help caregivers apply rational problem-solving techniques (see Chapter 3, this volume) to increasing self-care in order to improve their self-efficacy in this area of functioning. Some caregivers engage in pleasant activities on a regular basis, but the majority are hard pressed to remember the last time they did something enjoyable. Pleasant events are defined differently by each caregiver, so spending time in sessions brainstorming these favored activities is essential. Once the therapist and caregiver have identified activities that bring pleasure to the caregiver, they can work on increasing the time spent in rewarding pastimes.

In addition to interventions to improve self-care that take place outside the therapy session, the CFT therapist can also use time during therapy sessions to teach caregivers relaxation techniques. The goal of these additional strategies is to reduce stress and anxiety in the moment, and they can be used throughout the day. One example of a stress- and anxiety-reducing strategy is deep breathing, in which the caregiver consciously takes long, deep breaths and thinks calming thoughts. Other strategies for increasing mindfulness, ability to be present and experience emotion, and meditation are typically in the repertoire of mental health providers and can be applied with caregivers.

SOCIAL SELF-CARE

In addition to assessing and intervening to improve biological and psychological self-care, CFT therapists work with caregivers to enhance their social well-being. Caregivers can benefit greatly from finding and making time for meaningful social connections, such as friends and joyful family encounters. Going to work is not sufficient to meet a caregiver's needs for social interaction, although work contacts may be key members of a social network who would be missed if the caregiver quit work to remain at home with the care recipient. CFT therapists look broadly for the social connections that are relevant to a particular caregiver and invite caregivers to expand their definitions and experiences of social self-care.

Key questions include the following:

- Do you spend time with friends or in social activities?
- Do you enjoy these activities?
- Who and what agencies are in your support system?
- Are family conflicts contributing to stress, distress, and/or burden?
- Do you feel that you are managing tasks related to caregiving adequately?
- If not, what would help you to feel like you are doing a great job as a caregiver?

Individuals have varying needs for and interest in engaging in social interaction, but almost everyone needs some social connection. Social connections may be with family members, friends, colleagues, or others with similar interests, such as fellow bridge or golf club members. Caregivers, similarly, need to engage in multiple relationships outside of the caregiver–care recipient dyad. During later life, older adults' social networks become smaller, and they tend to focus on a few very close relationships rather than seeking out new and diverse people with whom to form relationships (Fung & Carstensen, 2004). During a period of caregiving when that role can become overloading, caregivers may be particularly uninterested in seeking novel social connections but need to be encouraged to connect at least with familiar social partners.

The CFT therapist assesses whether the caregivers' social contacts are satisfying and enriching. CFT therapists typically inquire about social interactions and social support during each session of therapy because, for many people, social opportunities are a key means of engaging in self-care, provided that those interactions are primarily positive and satisfying. Both family members and friends are valued members of social networks across the life span (Fiori, Antonucci, & Cortina, 2006). Therapists simply need to ensure that caregivers are maintaining connections within existing networks that are satisfying. Formal caregivers (e.g., therapist, rabbi or pastor, social worker) as well as informal supports (e.g., neighbors, friends) may be included in a caregiver's social support network, as long as the relationships provide the caregivers a measure of support and do not add to their burden or distress.

Further, the therapist works with the caregiver to increase pleasurable social activities, including time spent with close family members, friends, and other people in the caregivers' lives. Interventions to improve social interaction can take many forms and are tailored to meet the needs of individual caregivers. Some caregivers need more assistance with maintaining balance between spending time with the care recipient, taking time for self, and negotiating time to be with other family members and friends. Some caregivers need encouragement to seek out desired relationships and activities, and others need assistance with maintaining relationships, which can be accomplished through psychoeducation about social skills.

Caregivers often need to spend time interacting with other people who understand and can validate their experiences. Support groups may fulfill that need, but CFT therapists need to help caregivers determine (and teach them how to determine for themselves) whether they are being bogged down in other caregivers' negative reactions to caregiving. When caregivers truly feel supported in these types of groups, then they are likely fulfilling their purpose. Caregivers can also benefit from making new social connections with others who have experiences like theirs. Staff in support agencies, human resources staff at work, and other acquaintances may all be able to provide a sounding board for caregivers as they work through caregiving concerns. Being able to talk to others who are in a similar situation is a self-care activity in and of itself, and additionally, caregivers gain opportunities to learn from other caregivers about methods of interacting with their care recipients, family members, and virtual teams.

Like all humans, caregivers need a confidant (Weiss, 1973). If a caregiver is caring for a spouse who was previously the one to whom he or she confided, and if the care recipient has experienced functional losses that affect his or her understanding and sympathy toward the caregiver, the caregiver may have to establish a new pattern of interacting with friends or other family members in more intimate ways. Caregivers in this situation may also experience grief and loss associated with the decline in functioning of the care recipient and changes to his or her personality as a result.

In addition to increasing self-care activities related to the caregiving journey, caregivers simply need to find ways to play and have fun. For each caregiver, this will look different. It is not particularly important which pleasant activities the caregiver initiates or increases as long as he or she finds a way to spend some time doing something pleasant.

Caregivers who have not been to see a primary care physician in several years, who are regularly distressed about their situations, or who feel overwhelmed by the seemingly simple task of taking their care recipient to the doctor for a checkup very likely need to spend some time learning about the benefits of self-care to both themselves and the care recipient.

Integrating Findings Into a Self-Care Plan

The CFT therapist takes information about the caregiver's well-being, care recipient demands, and family context, as well as the stage of caregiving, and integrates this information into a care or treatment plan. Self-care strategies are based on prioritized goals set by the caregiver in terms of his or her most pressing needs. If health concerns are present, these likely take precedence over less urgent self-care activities, such as travelling for pleasure, because of the potential impact of a significant illness on both the caregiver and care recipient. When mental health concerns are present, the therapist determines whether the symptoms were present prior to the client initiating his or her role as a caregiver. The therapist might take different approaches with a client on the basis of whether the mental health concerns emerged in reaction to caregiving stress and burden or to long-standing diagnoses of mood, anxiety, or personality disorders. Further, information about the family context of caregiving and social support helps provide the therapist with avenues that the caregiver might take to enlist instrumental and other types of support from others.

Self-Care Resources and Activities

In the course of balancing the needs of caregiver and care recipient, many caregivers will need to learn to ask for help. The cultural value of independence and self-reliance makes it harder to ask for help than to keep pushing to do everything on one's own. Although early stages of caregiving may be manageable by one person alone, later stages of caregiving rarely can be handled alone. Thus, enlisting help from others is usually a skill that caregivers will need to develop over time. The extent to which a caregiver has requested help from formal and informal care providers can give the therapist an indication of the caregiver's awareness of the importance of self-care, knowledge of services, and willingness to access help. For example, a caregiver or care recipient may not have seen a physician if health insurance is lacking. In the U.S., language may be a barrier for some caregivers for whom English is not their first language. Caregivers also may have difficulty navigating complex health care systems so may access some but not all of the services needed. Informal care providers may not be accessible to caregivers who have not lived in their area for very long and to those who do not have large social or family networks in their geographical area. Enlisting help from formal and informal care providers may prove to be more difficult in some families than in others. Financial resources as well as ties to the community and family members have direct bearing on this aspect of caregiver self-care.

EXTERNAL RESOURCES

CFT therapists will find it useful to know at what level each family has already engaged service providers and whether the services that are currently in place are meeting the needs of the care recipient and the family. A family that has engaged the help of a neurologist, has been to the local Area Agency on Aging (AAA), and has begun looking into residential options for older adults is in a different place in their caregiving journey than the family that has not even consulted their primary care physician. Both of these families are functioning differently than the family that has had police or Adult Protective Services involved because of concerns about the health and safety of the care recipient. Some caregivers have already been working with another therapist in the community to improve mental health and may only be seeking CFT as a secondary and time-limited focus of treatment. On a checklist of locally available services, caregivers can quickly check those with which they have been in contact as a quick strategy for gathering information about the caregiver's support services. Although the problem-solving step of CFT (i.e., structuring care) would have helped calibrate care recipient needs with resources to meet them, at this point it is useful to review external services involvement again, but this time with an eye toward supporting the caregiver's well-being. The external resources available to caregivers of older adults include both formal and informal care providers.

Formal Systems of Support

Formal providers are those who are paid, such as physicians, medical specialists, neuropsychologists, as well as nursing assistants or personal care providers. Some personal care providers come to the family home and allow the primary caregiver to leave to engage in activities outside of the home, and others work on-site at residential or adult day-care facilities. When family members are unavailable or unable to assist with caregiving tasks, formal care providers should be considered. Paid care providers can be invited into the home for a few hours, or the care recipient can go to sites where providers are present during the day. In some cases, care recipients can even stay at a facility with care providers for a few days.

Respite care programs (e.g., adult day services) allow caregivers to enroll their care recipient for a few hours or all day in a day program and, if located in a residential setting, for several days at a time. Other respite services are provided in the home. The use of respite programs has been found to reduce actual caregiver time spent dealing with care recipient behavior problems as well as caregivers' perceptions of the care recipient exhibiting behavior problems overall (Gaugler et al., 2003; Gaugler & Zarit, 2001). Caregivers can and should be encouraged to access respite for their care recipients for periods of time when the caregiver can either focus on self-care activities, such as going to a football game with friends, or simply going grocery shopping for a few hours. When a caregiver wants to go out of town for a day or two, he or she can often arrange for a few overnight stays at a nearby nursing home. Facilities that offer respite can be accessed by plugging into one's local AAA and by working with geriatric care managers. Although care recipients might resist, the caregiver can be coached to go ahead and try respite for short and then longer periods of time on the premise that a caregiver will be able to provide a better quality of care if he or she takes time to care for his or her own needs in addition to the needs of the care recipient.

Many caregivers benefit from attending counseling and support groups (for reviews of therapy approaches and outcomes, see the American Psychological Association's caregiver website, http://www.apa.org/pi/about/publications/caregivers/index.aspx; Gallagher-Thompson & Coon, 2007; Pinquart & Sörensen, 2006). In many cases, support groups provide caregivers opportunities to learn that they are not alone, to increase the number of people in their support network, and to allow for the interchange of ideas related to caregiving problem-solving efforts. In some cases, however, caregivers may feel more stressed and worried about the future when hearing other caregivers' stories and may become caught up in shared depression with other caregivers.

Assistive technologies have also been found to be useful in managing the day-to-day demands of caregiving (Gitlin et al., 2003; Gitlin, Winter, & Dennis, 2010). Gitlin and colleagues taught caregivers to use several strategies of environmental modifications to enhance support to the care recipient, which relieved some of the burden felt by caregivers. Physical modifications of the environment included installation of safety equipment, such as grab bars in the shower and handrails around the home. Simple techniques included labeling items around the home and placing them in easy-to-access areas, the use of signs, and color contrasting. Making tasks simple and planning daily activities further adapt the environment to enhance care recipient functioning.

Geriatric care managers are excellent resources for caregivers in identifying evaluation and assessment resources and agencies and individuals that provide oversight and monitoring, and they are especially useful when family members cannot manage resource coordination because of distance, conflict within the family, or overwhelming other responsibilities. The National Association of Professional Geriatric Care Managers (http://www.caremanager.org) and National Academy of Certified Care Managers (http://www.naccm.net) provide listings of certified geriatric care managers. Geriatric care managers can link caregivers to local resources, and/or caregivers can search http://www.eldercare.gov to find the nearest AAA.

Funding for resources is available from various sources. Medicare and its supplemental insurances cover health care only, whereas private long-term-care insurance typically covers day care and residential services. Public funding supports other services, such as transportation, Meals on Wheels, and information/assistance phone lines.

Informal Systems of Support

Informal providers are identified within the personal network of friends, family members, and neighbors. Informal providers may include a good friend who listens on the phone after a stressful day or a neighbor who picks up a gallon of milk while she is at the store. Informal providers for most caregivers include family members who live close by. Caregivers likely examined options for having family members become involved in providing instrumental care and supportive functions to the caregiver during the role-structuring phase of CFT. Whatever collaboration between family members is happening needs to be monitored for ongoing stressors in that collaboration.

Most caregivers are embedded within a system of care that includes some level of support. In some families, multiple people may provide instrumental as well as supportive care roles, whereas in other families, the caregiver may be the only person living in the geographical area where the care recipient lives and requires care. In the latter situations, caregivers usually rely on others in their environments to support them. In one case, a husband may be caring for his wife, who is declining in both physical and cognitive functioning. Although he may not have asked for their help, his apartment managers have noticed that he is struggling with caring for his wife alone. The apartment managers offer to assist him with transferring his wife from their home to their car if only he will call when he needs assistance. Many people spontaneously make such informal support arrangements with their natural contacts in day-to-day life.

Family relationships are critical to self-care for two primary reasons. First is the fact that self-care includes making sure that the caregiving demands are manageable to the caregiver and family members may be an important source of instrumental support to caregivers who provide respite time for self-care. The second reason that family relationships are important is that self-care activities include addressing the social needs of caregivers, and for many people, their primary social contacts are their family members. Some caregivers may have several people in their families whom they consider sources of support, and others may have no one. For those who have no one in their families, the therapist may want to inquire about the possibility of working on improving a particular familial relationship in order to enhance the caregiver's feelings of well-being and to increase support from family members. On the other hand, if most of the relationships between the caregiver's family members have been cut off, and if the caregiver does not believe that reconciliation is possible, then focusing self-care interventions on finding other sources of social support might be most beneficial.

Knowing who might be available to provide assistance is only the first step in working toward asking for help. A family member may live close by, be retired, and have free time available to help, and the caregiver may still experience difficulty asking that family member for help. Determining what is getting in the way of the caregiver talking with that person about getting involved in caregiving tasks will help the therapist to know whether it is realistic to involve that particular family member in the caregiving process.

Families with weak or strained emotional bonds can be disappointed or frustrated when seeking assistance from family members. In other words, asking for help may not lead to help received or may lead to assistance with tasks that arrives without warm communication or kind motivations. Long-term histories of bitter conflicted relationships are unlikely to produce supportive assistance during caregiving periods. However, a caregiver may still be able to obtain a specific piece of assistance from a family member who harbors no warm fuzzy feelings about giving it. Sometimes, caregivers need to learn to accept what is available within the family in order to balance the caregiver's self-care needs with the tasks that need to be done. Even if it is very limited in emotional value or comes with some prickly communication, the "gift" from an emotionally unavailable family member may be useful because it frees up time for self-care.

CFT therapists must assess the familial relationships prior to encouraging increased interaction among family members, in particular interaction that is focused on enlisting support. A caregiver's sense of dread about asking for help must be understood well before proceeding to plan such a request. Dread may reflect a generalized reluctance to ask for help. It may also be informed by a long history of communication that the therapist needs to understand.

Families that are distant but not conflicted may have potential for engagement if information is shared thoughtfully. Ideally, a request for help is not loaded with assignments of guilt to the other for not having already pitched in. Caregivers need to be able to ask using clear "I" statements, with some role-playing to ensure that they can articulate their needs without introducing emotionally loaded language.

Families with a long history of conflict are unlikely to respond with empathy for the caregiver's situation, so they may need to hear the request more factually, appealing to their bond with the care recipient more than the bond with caregiver as motivation to engage. Caregivers asking a family member with whom there is a long history of conflict need to be prepared to ask in very factual ways and to have thought through how they want to address all possible responses. Therapists can help caregivers clarify expectations, lowering them to a level that seems realistic given the family history. Rather than focusing on what others "could be doing but aren't," the caregiver can be oriented to the benefits of obtaining some assistance at a time of high stress.

INTERNAL RESOURCES

Internal needs and assets are cognitive, emotional, and spiritual resources that support self-care during caregiving. Examples include empowering the caregiver to attend to relational needs, teaching the caregiver to reframe the care recipient's problem behaviors, and increasing assertiveness skills when working with family members and community agencies (S. H. Jones, 2007). We discuss several domains of internal resources that arise commonly when working with caregivers on self-care.

Values About Prioritizing Self-Care

Clients' values about prioritizing self-care in the context of caring for another are likely to influence their self-care decisions. Before being in a position to help guide a caregiver into balancing care for self and others, the caregiver's values and orientation to caregiving itself needs to be assessed. Caregivers fall along a continuum ranging from minimalist approaches to care to super helpful. For example, one caregiver may tend to do everything for her spouse, even though he is still capable of doing many things for himself. Another caregiver may tend not to do things for her husband, even in light of information that suggests he is not capable of completing those tasks himself (see the example in Exhibit 6.2).

Caregivers may have several reasons for jumping in to do something for their care recipient or for not wanting to step in. Exploring the

EXHIBIT 6.2

Mr. Wright (Continued)

Mr. Wright finds it difficult to strike a balance between his roles as a son, husband, and father, not to mention his responsibilities at work. His wife now undergoes chemotherapy every third week, and for about a week after each treatment, she feels tired, worn down, and mildly sick to her stomach. She takes about 3 days off from work every time she undergoes chemotherapy treatment, which is beginning to put some financial strain on their family. Mr. Wright reports that everyone in the family is concerned about Mrs. Wright's health, especially their daughter. Her grades are suffering because she has picked up a part-time job to help her parents out, and she also finds herself worrying and feeling scared about her mother's well-being. Mr. Wright also indicates that he is having difficulty sleeping and that his appetite has decreased. He thought that he was managing all of his roles well enough, but last week he "about lost it" when his mother fell and broke her wrist while she was fixing lunch for herself and her husband.

In Mr. Wright's family, his daughter could potentially spend some extra time with her grandparents during the evenings, cooking for them and assisting them with household tasks as needed. Mr. Wright might also be able to call on his son for help at times, which could potentially strengthen their relationship. Furthermore, Mr. Wright might be encouraged to call his sister, who lives in another state, to talk about their parents, to seek advice, and to obtain emotional support from her. He may want to ask her to share costs of paid instrumental care.

reasons behind their decisions will help the therapist to work toward changing the caregiver's attitudes when necessary. Overinvolved caregivers will face challenges in self-care because their time is devoted to caring for the other; underinvolved caregivers may happily engage in self-care while denying the risk to the care recipient who truly needs help from that person or another caregiver.

Many caregivers report feeling guilty about taking time away from the care recipient in order to complete self-care strategies, and this guilt should be explored and normalized in session. Spouses in particular struggle with allocating time for themselves, away from their loved ones with whom they previously shared their pleasant activities. Some caregivers may identify very closely with the caregiving role and find it difficult to step into other roles, such as becoming one who exercises, one who plays bridge with friends, or one who goes on vacation. These caregivers often derive meaning and self-esteem from their time spent engaged in caregiving activities, which can be a valuable part of the caregiving experience. However, taken to the extreme, the overly dedicated caregiver may feel that she is worthless if she is not doing something for someone else. In cases such as these, the CFT therapist must find the root of those beliefs within the caregiver and use cognitive–behavioral therapy techniques to address poor self-esteem, lack of self-worth, and self-sabotage when they are present (A. T. Beck & Alford, 2009; Burns, 1999).

Time Management

Key to balancing time spent on giving care with time spent on self is time management. Without explicit plans, good intentions rarely result in action. Consider the oft-cited analogy of small and large rocks being placed in a jar. If a pile of small rocks is poured in first, there is room for only a few of the large rocks. But if the large rocks are placed in first, the small rocks can sift down around the large ones, filling the jar with little airspace left over. Caregivers can be encouraged to schedule their self-care priorities first and let the small daily caregiving tasks fall around them.

CFT or other formal supportive services can be considered self-care activities that allow the caregiver to debrief each week with a person who is supportive and understanding. Sometimes, engaging in therapy is the only self-care activity in which a caregiver can conceive of participating initially. A goal of the self-care work of CFT may be to build an appropriate range of activities that will sustain well-being long after an episode of CFT is completed.

The freedom to engage in self-care activities will wax and wane throughout the course of caregivers' journeys. As care recipients' needs increase for periods of time, caregivers may have to reduce time spent focusing on themselves, and as pressures decrease, self-care activities can again be instituted.

Problem Solving for Specific Stressors

Chapter 3 details the use of the problem-solving approach (D'Zurilla, Nezu, & Maydeu-Olivares, 2004) in CFT on behalf of the care recipient; those same skills are relevant to overcoming barriers to self-care. As a review, the steps of problem solving involve approaching problems from a positive orientation, naming the problem in specific terms, brainstorming solutions to the problem, weighing the pros and cons of the possible solutions, trying a solution, and then evaluating whether the chosen solution worked. These steps can be used to choose and implement a self-care approach.

The therapist and caregiver work together on problem-solving skills related to setting priorities. For example, which problem needs to be tackled first—the caregiver's need for more sleep or her daughter's ongoing requests to care for her grandchild when she does not have the energy to babysit? The therapist can also help the caregiver to set small, realistic goals and then to offer praise when the caregiver accomplishes those goals.

When brainstorming personal goals for change, the CFT therapist and caregiver should consider both the advantages and disadvantages of making change. It is also useful to consider what strategies have worked in the past as well as current and possible future obstacles that the caregiver might encounter. As with all problem-solving work, homework can be assigned to the caregiver that guides him or her through steps in the process outside of sessions. Activities that promote health and/or are enjoyable are good candidates for personal goals related to self-care.

Possible health maintenance activities to consider include the following:

- maintaining a proper diet,
- adequate amount of sleep,
- exercise,
- regular medical physicals, and
- maintaining hygiene and grooming.

Possible pleasurable activities to consider include the following:

- exercise,
- reading or puzzles,
- movies and museums,
- visiting with friends, and
- personal hobbies.

Relational self-care activities might include addressing interpersonal strains that come about during the caregiving journey. Such strains have great potential to add to the feelings of stress and burden experienced by caregivers. Thus, CFT therapists can help caregivers work on improving their relationships during the caregiving process.

Once caregivers choose their goals, the therapist may want to shape the goals to be as specific as possible. A timeline for achieving goals may also keep the caregiver focused on action. It is important to check in with a client to ensure that goals are realistic and are not perceived as an additional burden.

Assessing Outcomes and Modifying When Necessary

The objective of assessing outcomes is to evaluate how the self-care process is changing and hopefully succeeding. Sheets for tracking the frequency of self-care activities are good resources. Reviewing these forms in session can initiate discussions surrounding what strategies have worked well for the client, what strategies have not been successful, and how the overall process of change has felt to the caregiver. Successfully working through self-care goals would include setting and maintaining self-care strategies by reducing symptoms of physical, psychological, or social strain and burden.

Almost any caregiver could benefit from time spent improving functioning in multiple areas, but it is unrealistic to work on several at one time. Particularly while providing care for another, there simply is not enough time and energy to tackle many at once. Therefore, CFT therapists must prioritize self-care strategies that are most necessary at any given time and target interventions toward those.

Self-Efficacy

Self-efficacy pertains to how an individual views his or her capacity to implement specific actions to achieve desirable outcomes (Bandura, 1977). For example, a caregiver with high self-efficacy for caregiving would believe that he has the skills and knowledge to arrange appointments and meals along with all of the other tasks associated with caregiving. Further, a caregiver with very high self-efficacy would tend to remain in the caregiving role through the stages of illness of the care recipient, continuing to believe that he was capable of handling anything that might come his way. Another aspect of self-efficacy related to caregiving is the belief that one has the ability to manage the stressors and sense of burden that accompany the caregiving journey. It stands to reason that a person who has less self-efficacy related to caregiving and, in particular, to self-care, would be less likely to be successful in attempts to maintain self-care (Zeiss, Gallagher-Thompson, Lovett, Rose, & McKibbin, 1999). Caregivers with low self-efficacy related to self-care may not believe that they can make changes in their routines, such as make time to exercise, cook new recipes, or develop a new friendship, to promote self-care. Challenging these beliefs and encouraging caregivers to begin to establish their self-efficacy through problem solving (see Chapter 3) are strategies CFT therapists can use.

Caregiving self-efficacy has a positive impact on caregivers' coping and can decrease depression, distress, and burden (Zeiss et al., 1999). Zeiss et al. (1999) developed scales to test caregivers' self-efficacy in terms of self-care and problem solving, and they found that out of 10 self-care strategies, the caregivers felt strongly (ratings of 70% or above) that they could accomplish the following self-care tasks: having a positive phone conversation, spending time engaging in their own hobbies, getting out of the house without the care recipient, sharing their personal feelings, and keeping a positive attitude. However, caregivers were not certain that they could engage in a pleasant activity with the care recipient, get at least 7 hours of sleep a night, share their feelings at least once a week, or spend an hour a week doing something they enjoyed. Caregivers had difficulty believing they could accomplish the more specific goals that required the caregiver to commit to completing a self-care activity on a daily or weekly basis.

In terms of problem solving, the caregivers rated the four items of naming a problem specifically, listing solutions, choosing the best solution, and carrying out the plan between 68.9% and 76.7%, relatively high indicators of self-efficacy, in terms of their confidence that they could complete these tasks. Additionally, Zeiss et al. (1999) found that higher ratings of self-care and problem-solving self-efficacy were related to lower reports of depression and burden.

Given the findings of Zeiss et al. (1999), a CFT therapist must look for opportunities to improve caregivers' feelings of self-efficacy related self-care and problem solving. As caregivers go through the steps of problem solving and increasing self-care activities, their perceptions of their self-efficacy are likely to increase over time. CFT therapists should be ready to look for the positive outcomes in any situation and to reflect those back to the caregiver, modeling positive thinking whenever possible. For example, even when an attempt to improve self-care does not work out as planned, the therapist can state to the caregiver that it took courage to try something new. Further, helping the caregiver to think ahead about problems that could arise when trying new approaches to caregiving and self-care activities might decrease the number of strategies he or she attempts before finding one that will be successful.

Addressing Barriers

Many caregivers insist on placing the care recipients' needs ahead of their own. They hesitate to spend time with friends and family members; they also decrease time spent alone doing things they always enjoyed and resist suggestions about taking a break from caregiving, even for a few hours. Frequently, these caregivers feel guilty about taking care of their own needs when they see that their care recipient is declining in health. Others fear and resist change as a general approach to difficult situations in their lives. As dedicated as these caregivers often are, their refusal to attend to their own physical, psychological, and social needs actually impedes the caregiving process. Caregivers stopped from engaging in self-care by guilt can easily become worn down and physically sick and often experience higher levels of stress and burden associated with caregiving. Alternatively, self-care assists caregivers in feeling more energetic, fulfilled in multiple domains of their lives, and efficacious in regard to caregiving.

ENHANCING URGENCY

Just as CFT often enhances a sense of urgency to clarify the consequences of poor elder care (e.g., what would happen if mother got in a bad car accident because no one was brave enough to confront her about her declining driving abilities?; see Chapter 4), CFT also enhances urgency to mobilize self-care by clarifying the consequences of poor self-care. Unfortunately, many caregivers place self-care at the very lowest position on their priority list. They mistakenly believe that the care recipient's (and often everyone else's) needs absolutely must be taken care of before their own. These caregivers run the very high risk of becoming physically ill or injured and in some cases risk death because of extremely poor self-care. Therefore, therapists realize that the only way to help these caregivers to stop neglecting their own needs is to shock them into thinking about what would happen if they did suddenly become incapacitated—what if they were hit by a bus and sent to the hospital in a coma, unable to call in help from anyone else or even notify someone that their care recipient was left home alone while they ran to the store?

Therapists at the CU Aging Center affectionately refer to their most directive intervention to engage caregivers in prioritizing self-care as the "2 × 4." This metaphor implies that the client feels a bit stunned by the impact of the intervention that has metaphorically whopped him or her upside the head. The CFT therapist instructs the caregiver to use a visual exercise that walks the caregiver through an imaginary scenario in which he or she is incapacitated and unable to take care of the care recipient (e.g., in a hospital emergency room unable to speak, in a postoperative recovery room after surgery). During the visualization exercise, the caregiver is asked to think about where his or her loved one is, what level of risk is present, and whether anyone would know to check on the care recipient. The purpose of this exercise is to help the caregiver recognize the incredible importance of self-care on the future well-being of the care recipient and the value of sharing caregiving responsibilities at least to the extent that someone else would know how to fill in for the caregiver during a period of absence. In most cases, this visualization 2 × 4 can cause a reluctant caregiver to pause for a moment and consider, usually, two things: (a) I need a back-up emergency plan in case something happens to me, and (b) I need to start taking better care of myself.

SELF-VALUING

CFT therapists help caregivers to develop a clear rationale for why self-care is critical to both the caregiver and care recipient. The rationale addresses inner barriers such as thoughts that "I am not worth it" and "What will others think if I spend time on myself?"

CFT therapists spend time reframing caregivers' thoughts about themselves, focusing on helping them accept that their lives have value, just as their care recipients' lives are valuable. Some caregivers might benefit from hearing stories or analogies about parents of children with lifelong disabilities. When imagining caring for a person with disabilities across the life span, a caregiver is likely to accept that self-care would be essential in order for the parent to sustain caregiving for such a long period of time. In essence, caregivers of older adults may also spend many years engaged in caregiving, so drawing this parallel can help caregivers understand the need for self-care to sustain their caregiving efforts over time.

Some caregivers may experience a sense of shame about domains of life in which they have not engaged in good self-care across their life span. Weight management, long-term panic disorder, and poor assertiveness skills are just a few examples of physical, psychological, and social arenas in which caregivers may want help changing lifelong poor self-care habits. Therapists who work with midlife and older adults become accustomed to telling clients that it is never too late to begin addressing areas in which they hope to make change.

Caregivers with limited financial resources may argue that they are unable to engage in self-care activities because there is not enough money to care for both the care recipient and themselves. CFT therapists may hear many statements such as, "I can't just go buy a gym membership, new sneakers, or fresh fruit." In such instances, the therapist has many options, including asking the caregiver to generate a list of self-care activities that are free, providing the caregiver with information about free or low-cost local resources and asking caregivers to examine their finances to determine what resources might realistically be allocated to self-care activities.

One of the most universal arguments caregivers give for avoiding self-care activities, especially those that are pleasant, is that it is not OK for them to have fun or joy in their lives without the care recipient. Some experience shame about taking time away from their care recipients, especially spouses, and doing fun activities in which the other spouse cannot participate. Some caregivers worry what their friends and family members will think if they do not spend all of their time with the care recipient and wonder how to explain to others (including the care recipient) that self-care is a new priority to them. Caregivers who provide in-home care will need to come up with ways of responding to the care recipient's questions about activities outside the home (e.g., "Where are you going, and why can't I come?"). Therapists need to role-play such scenarios until the caregiver feels capable of responding in a way that has integrity. Coaching in simple responses followed by a quick exit is very helpful. Caregivers often need help dealing with the guilt they feel when walking out the door of the home or residential facility to live some piece of their lives that the care recipient cannot share. Some caregivers also know that they may realistically need to address their fears that others will critique them for their "selfishness," and therapists can help guide caregivers through these conversations in role-playing exercises.

Ultimately, CFT therapists want to convey to caregivers that "caring for me is critical to us both." When caregivers resist the idea of self-care, therapists can use the common reminder that when flying on an airplane, passengers are directed to place their own oxygen mask on their face before helping the person sitting next to them. The implied message is that if people do not take care of themselves, they will not be capable of caring for someone else.

PRAGMATICS

Each caregiver's journey is different, so interventions to address self-care must be tailored to the specific needs of the caregiver, the care recipient, and the individual circumstances of each case. For example, a therapist may be tempted to dive into helping a client create a new meal plan and exercise routine, but this may not be the best place to begin. Considering the effects of these changes on the caregiver, the care recipient, and other family members prior to developing a plan may go a long way toward increasing the likelihood of the plan's success. Indeed, caregivers often live in a social context in which other people have a powerful influence over the their self-care activities.

Staggering self-care goals over time to ensure that they are manageable is important and indicates respect for the time involved in caregiving tasks and the complexity of each caregiver's day-to-day routine. Also, emphasizing the benefits of small changes will encourage the caregiver to continue taking small steps over time that eventually will lead to better overall well-being. Clients do not always notice the benefits of gradual changes. Simple systems for tracking the desirable outcomes offer clear feedback for both client and therapist that the strategy being used is working, or not (see the example in Exhibit 6.3).

Caregivers manifest their stress in diverse ways. For example, some will notice tension in their shoulders while others have headaches, and yet others yell at the people closest to them when they are overwhelmed with their lives. CFT therapists teach their clients to become familiar with their own patterns of exhibiting stress so that caregivers can eventually gain a sense of control over their reactions. At the first signs of stress, caregivers can learn to respond by taking steps to relax, doing something positive for themselves, and seeking help when needed.

In each caregiving situation, the CFT therapist will want to identify the best practice of self-care for this particular person in this particular family. Once an area of functioning is named as a priority, the therapist and caregiver work together to structure an exact plan for implementing

EXHIBIT 6.3

Consuela

Consuela is a 70-year-old caregiver for her husband, Roberto, who had a stroke about 1 year ago. Roberto experiences some difficulty with his speech, and he becomes disoriented in crowds and when his routine is disrupted. Consuela has Type 2 diabetes and is overweight for her small stature. In addition to caring for her husband, she is raising their 10-year-old grandson, Jesse, whose parents were killed in a car accident several years ago. Consuela emphasizes during CFT sessions that for the most part, she feels comfortable caring for Roberto and Jesse, but she struggles with finding respite when she needs to attend meetings for Jesse at his school. Although she has two daughters who live nearby who always ask her how they can help, she tries not to overburden them because they have busy lives and families of their own. In addition to finding child care for Jesse, Consuela would also like to focus on her diet and exercise, but she feels nervous about changing the food options available in her household—the men may not agree with the new menu—and she is not sure where to begin with an exercise routine. Consuela noted in her last session that she primarily struggles with feeling tired in the afternoon most days, and she also reported that she feels sad, weary, and sometimes angry in the late evenings. She was unsure why she feels angry, but these feelings were concerning to her because she indicated that she had always been a pretty relaxed and easygoing person earlier in her life.

After discussing her options with her therapist, Consuela decided to consult her physician about exercises that would be safe for her to try in order to begin making improvements in her health. She also decided to begin adding more green, leafy salads to her existing diet so that Roberto and Jesse would be able to slowly adjust to some healthy lifestyle changes. Consuela also found a senior center located near a YMCA in her community. She could take her husband to the senior center for an hour while she went next door to the pool to swim. Much to her surprise, she found that Roberto was happy and engaged at the senior center for short periods of time, so she was able to take him there on the occasions when she needed to meet with Jesse's teachers at school. By using these strategies, Consuela realized that in making a very small change, she could feel successful immediately (at least in one domain of self-care), while it might take some time for her to notice the effects of her initial exercise routine.

The therapist working with Consuela encouraged her to continue focusing on her physical health and addressing stressful situations that she encountered in caring for her grandson. They decided together that after a few months of this routine, Consuela would try to begin spending one evening every other week with some of her friends from church.

In addition to using more than one strategy to begin to improve her self-care, her therapist helped her to create a simple data tracking form to track her new behaviors; a few health markers (e.g., weight, energy level, blood sugar levels, need for insulin); and a few mood, stress, and coping outcomes. The therapist tailored the data tracking forms to address the specific behaviors Consuela was working on as well as the bothersome feelings that Consuela had experienced prior to beginning the self-care changes. The therapist also included space for Consuela to indicate any other noticeable emotional or physical responses to the changes she was making.

Using data tracking, both the therapist and Consuela could note where progress was and was not occurring. New self-care goals could be created as success with each previous goal reached a plateau. Over time, Consuela was able to notice a marked improvement in her energy level and mood, and by looking at her tracking forms, she was able to connect the improvements directly to the changes she had made in her behaviors. She noticed that when she didn't

(continued)

EXHIBIT 6.3 (Continued)

make it to the YMCA for a few of her swimming sessions, her mood worsened. Feelings of anger, although infrequent, were persistent despite the changes she had made. Consuela and her therapist decided that they would next try to focus on uncovering where the feeling of anger originated.

After several months of therapy, Consuela realized that her anger stemmed from her husband's inability to talk with her to help her process the aspects of her life she found difficult. In the past, he had always been a sounding board for her, and she had really needed his advice when dealing with upsets between her and her friends; when Jesse needed a man's guidance; and when she was feeling sad about the death of Jesse's parents, her daughter and son-in-law. The absence of her husband as a confidant increased her feelings of burden, which usually resulted in her storming around the house in a huff. Consuela said that she usually did not yell at her family members, but she frequently felt like it, after which she would dissolve into tears. During these times, she felt alone and frightened.

Working with her therapist, Consuela identified the first sign of trouble as being less energetic than usual, with intermittent bouts of irritability. If she scheduled an evening with a good friend or with one of her daughters during the first week when she began feeling tired, irritable, and sad, she could ward off the more intense feelings of anger that had developed over the past several months. She and her best friend made an agreement that they could call each other to debrief any time and that they would make sure to spend time out together at least once a month. Consuela learned that she could control symptoms that in the past felt overwhelming and baffling to her by taking time to relax and talk with a close family member or friend.

---

the self-care activity. The caregiver will need to take into account the time, money, and other resources required for the activity because any of these may function as barriers to success. Some caregivers benefit tremendously from enlisting a self-care buddy who can both provide support and add joy to self-care activities. A self-care buddy might also provide accountability for the caregiver's commitment to self-care, or this role might be performed by the therapist in the short term or a family member or friend over the long term.

Although some self-care activities are very physical and active, such as engaging in exercise and social activities, others involve centering time, such as journaling, meditating, and prayer. Caregivers may find that these activities help them stay on track with their personal priorities while also focusing on caregiving activities.

Regardless of the type of self-care activity, the CFT therapist can help the caregiver anticipate backsliding. Whether a person is a caregiver or not, we all go through times in life when self-care is more or less of a priority, and it is inevitable that we "blow it" when making difficult changes to improve our own well-being. CFT therapists can help prevent caregivers from becoming completely derailed by asking them to think about how to recover and get back on track when self-care takes a backseat to other responsibilities.

Conclusion

Self-care is another of those critical rubber-hits-the-road points in CFT. Similar to naming and role structuring in the size of the task and the magnitude of challenges to implementing good solutions, self-care is considered one of the three core processes of CFT. The ultimate goal of the therapist is to ensure that the caregiver is taking care of himself or herself while attending to the needs of the care recipient and also keeping in mind the needs of other family members. Self-care is needed in all domains of the biopsychosocial model, involving resources that are external as well as internal to the caregiver. The history of the person's efforts at self-care and the family system's rules about self-care are both salient and important here. Shame, guilt, and fear about attempting self-care are potent barriers to success in balancing care for self and other, as are limited resources. All must be worked through thoughtfully and carefully because self-care is easier to imagine than to implement. The care structures established in earlier phases of CFT may need to be revised to provide stronger support for the caregiver to balance self-care and care for others. At times, caregivers' attitudes toward self-care need to be modified, and in most cases, caregivers need to hear that self-care is important to the well-being of both the caregiver and the care recipient.

Widening the Lens and Anticipating the Future

7

The final steps of CFT involve taking a step back to get the widest possible view of the family's functioning and to look forward in anticipation of future transitions in care recipient functioning that will require another round of changes for the family. This chapter provides a rationale for looking broadly and looking forward before ending an episode of work with the caregiver(s). Both processes offer an opportunity for the caregiver to consider conditions under which the new caregiving structure will destabilize. Even if the structure created during caregiver family therapy (CFT) is perfectly suited to the needs of both care recipient and caregiver, the family is a system with many members whose needs also must be met. Furthermore, the best caregiving structure in the world will not remain stable forever—something or someone in the family will change. The care receiver's chronic disease is highly likely to advance over time, whether slowly or in crisis events, requiring a new cycle of adaptation of the caregiving structure. The caregiver's functioning may change

DOI: 10.1037/13943-007
Caregiver Family Therapy: Empowering Families to Meet the Challenges of Aging,
by S. H. Qualls and A. A. Williams

as well. This chapter offers a rationale, framework, and strategies for pausing at the end of an episode of CFT to consider the broader and future picture (case descriptions of this stage elaborated in Chapter 8).

Rationale for Widening the Lens to View the Broader Family System

The systems in which we live our lives contain many people who rely on us for various services and functions. The interconnectedness of units within a system, or people within a family, means that movements we make toward one commitment constrain our resources in another direction. When we establish a caregiving structure involving commitment to the care recipient, we are taking energy and focus from other family members who may truly need us.

Our family systems orientation draws us to give careful consideration to the broader systemic impact of the structures we so carefully help caregivers negotiate in the earlier steps of CFT. The sustainability of any caregiving situation relies on the stability of the family structures and processes the caregiver has put into place. If family members' needs are not being met in familiar ways, innovative approaches to meeting those needs will emerge. Some of them may have a big price for the family.

Who Is Impacted by the Caregiving Role?

The primary caregiver's genogram offers a great starting point for widening the lens. Although a genogram was likely developed very early in the CFT process, it is possible that the initial genogram revolved around the care recipient and lacks the information to widen the focus around the caregiver now. In the latter case, the caregiver may need to develop a genogram of his or her own family in order to look through a wide lens at the impact of caregiving in his or her life.

The family members who are mapped onto the caregiver's genogram are all potentially impacted by the new roles implemented by the caregiver(s). Caregivers who are parents need to review the extent to which resources needed by their children have become less (or more) available, and caregivers who are married or partnered need to do the same for the spouse or partner (see the example in Exhibit 7.1).

EXHIBIT 7.1

Henry

Henry always had a close and loving relationship with his wife, Andrea, and a strong bond with their son, James (19), who lives in a city a few hours away. Despite his misgivings, Henry brought his mother to live with them from out of state when her Alzheimer's disease progressed to a point at which she could no longer live independently. Henry's mother was a safety risk. She had severely impaired memory, would spend hours on end staring out the window and occasionally had angry outbursts. She was unsafe alone because she would forget to turn off the stove or to bathe properly. Caring for her was time consuming. Most of her time needed to be structured for her, and she required ongoing prompting to finish simple tasks, such as dressing and eating. Henry had never had a positive relationship with his mother and was openly resentful about her moving in. He acknowledged that her living with him and his wife was a temporary solution while his mother's finances were settled. Henry's mother lived with him and his wife for nearly a year, during which James was diagnosed with testicular cancer and a litany of other health problems. James lost his job and health insurance and was impoverished by medical bills. Henry expressed a desire to help James financially and, more important, to spend more time with him, but felt he this was impossible. Because of the costs of caring for his mother and the constant level of supervision she required, Henry was unable to adequately support James (Anderson et al., 2008).

Henry and his son suffered because of the commitment Henry made to the care of his mother. Henry had created a viable approach to meeting his mother's needs that did not excessively burden him until it became clear that his commitment to her was costing his son. Although Henry could not have anticipated that James's needs would change so dramatically because of his unfolding health crisis, he certainly had a strong desire to respond to his son's needs.

Henry became more depressed and anxious as he watched his son struggle without his help. His voice took on an impatient edge when he cared for his mother's needs. His wife began to stay away from home longer hours after work to avoid the tension at home, increasing her involvement in church and clubs. Henry started to feel isolated and burdened in a way he had not for the past year when he cared for his mother. The therapist helped him examine the impact of his caregiving on those he loved and to revisit his decision to provide all of his mother's care himself. Together Henry and his therapist explored alternative strategies for caring for her, ultimately choosing to move her to a small assisted living residence a few blocks away from his home. He worked with the facility to get her qualified for Medicaid, which paid for the placement in full, leaving Henry's personal resources available to share with James. James moved back home into the bedroom suite that Henry had prepared for his mother, affording James independence and the privacy of a small apartment. Henry invited his wife into a session to discuss the impact of the care needs of both his mother and James on their marriage. Widening the lens was initially quite threatening to Henry but ended up likely saving his marriage as well as enriching his relationship with his son.

Note. From *The Aging Families and Caregiver Program: A Guide to Caregiver Family Therapy,* by L. Anderson, S. Horning, A. June, K. Kane, M. Marty, R. Pepin, and C. Vair, 2008, Unpublished manuscript. Copyright 2008 by L. Anderson, S. Horning, A. June, K. Kane, M. Marty, R. Pepin, and C. Vair. Reprinted with permission.

Siblings may be affected by the additional duties someone has embraced as caregiver. The range of potentially impacted relationships is quite broad within the family. Certainly, nonfamilial roles are also quite likely to be affected, but the focus of CFT is on *family* by definition.

Has Caregiving Increased or Decreased the Family's Resources?

Once it is clear who might be affected by caregiving, how this may happen can be investigated. A first question relates to the losses that might be experienced by those close to the caregiver because of his or her additional caregiving roles. What time, energy, nurturance, problem solving, attention, or care has been shifted from close family members to the care recipient? The loss may or may not impact development, depending on whether the caregiver was previously supplying a key condition for development. On the other hand, the emergence of behavior problems, underperformance in any aspect of biopsychosocial functioning, or a shift in mood or other well-being indicators may be the indicator that individual developmental needs are not being met. Individual development requires environmental contexts (including physical, social, and psychological) that offer both stimulation and support. Development proceeds effectively when the conditions to support it are intact, but it is thwarted when those conditions are removed. Marriages need time invested in shared pleasant activities in order to withstand the stresses of daily life that draw individuals apart. Adolescents who are independent in many aspects of self-care need time with parents for guidance, driver training, homework check-in accountability, and career planning, in addition to nurturance for their fragile, developing egos. A caregiver's daughter who has her first baby needs to feel supported and likely needs input on care strategies as she adjusts to this new role, and a parent is a typical source of that support. A key focus, then, is how the caregiver's current role(s) may reduce resources that were supportive of development in other family members.

A second question is how the caregiver's new role(s) may add resources to the family. Some individuals are empowered by the caregiving roles, growing into more effective and confident people. When this occurs, other family members may actually gain from the caregiver's expanded capacity to function (see the example in Exhibit 7.2). Others may also experience positive gain from someone's commitment to caregiving if it redirects the attention of hypervigilant family members away from those whose development may otherwise have been smothered.

EXHIBIT 7.2

Suzie

Suzie has served as the local caregiver for her neighbor, John, for the past 3 years. His family, whose members are geographically dispersed, gratefully welcomed her into the "family" for this purpose. John's children send her funds to buy his holiday gifts as well as clothes and other supplies when needed. She refuses money to pay for her time or food supplies when she cooks for him. The caregiving situation is stable for the moment, now that caregiver family therapy (CFT) has helped her balance her commitments to John with services from a home health agency. Early in CFT, she helped create John's genogram, which illuminated options for renegotiating her role with other members of John's family, even though they all live at a distance. Now, it is time to revisit Suzie's family responsibilities to make sure that the caregiving role she embraces with John can be sustained without cost to others in her family. Suzie and the CFT therapist constructed a genogram of her family when it was time to look at her role load in the last review point of the CFT cycle. Suzie now pulls that back out for review.

Suzie is a single woman who never married or had children and has few responsibilities within her own family. Her caregiving relationship to John has increased her confidence that she could handle caring for another person day in and day out. Secretly, she had always questioned whether she was too selfish to marry or to have children. She now knows that she can maintain a commitment with joy, appreciating the structure it has added to her evenings and weekends. Her sister's family, however, misses her monthly visits to their home a few hours away for long weekends, and she notices that her nieces and nephews are less talkative with her on the telephone. The wider lens has helped her review the impact of her choices to forego those trips in order to care for John. On reflection, she checks back with John's family about alternative weekend care options that would free her to resume her monthly visits with her sister's family. They are happy to fund additional home health services on the weekend.

Suzie's sister is thrilled that Suzie is back visiting regularly and quite surprised to find that her sister is so much more comfortable doing care tasks for the children. Previously, Aunt Suzie was a source of fun, but she offered little assistance with practical aspects of child care. Suzie now steps in with confidence to give baths, dress the kids for bed, prepare meals, and enforce bedtime rules. The children have their fun Aunt Suzie back, with even more nurturance contact as she helps with practical child care as well as fun outings.

Suzie's sister adapts quickly to the expanded skills and confidence her sister brings to the family! Suzie is now ready to offer her sister and brother-in-law a weekend away while she babysits, an offer she would have not felt confident to offer previously. Suzie and her sister also share more detailed conversations about the dilemmas of child rearing than either would have broached previously. Although their parents are too young to need assistance, they also occasionally discuss future scenarios and how they would like to handle them. Their conversations simply are more intimate than they have been in years.

Key questions to ask the caregiver include the following:

▪ Given the caregiving tasks the client must do, what times of day and what levels of energy are being diverted away from the previous lifestyle?

▪ Which family members are likely to be impacted by the client's caregiving responsibilities?

▪ How is each one likely to be affected positively? Negatively?

- Where would you expect family members to be developmentally at this point?
- Have any family members shown a regression in development (behavior problems, underperformance, mood problems, or other indicators of poor well-being)?
- What are some changes in relationships? What are the repercussions?
- How have relational priorities shifted?
- How have those affected by the client's investment in caregiving adapted, positively and negatively?
- What will happen if these adaptations extend for a long period of time?

The CFT therapist may not be able to help the primary caregiver balance the needs of all family members on his or her own but may look to adding secondary caregiving resources to balance unmet needs. The role of the CFT therapist is to inquire about the reverberations of caregiving for other family members and invite the client to think about how caregiving has created challenges and opportunities that affect a broader range of people than just the primary caregivers. Strategies for filling gaps to support other members' development may take the caregiver client back to the problem-solving stage of CFT to review other options for meeting the care recipient's needs that would demand less of one person. Alternatively, the caregiver client may be able to identify other strategies for meeting needs of the other family members, including recognizing that they have adapted in their own ways to having less of the caregiver's time and energy.

How Have Others Adapted to the Caregiver's New Roles?

As the caregiver's role shifts reverberate throughout the family system, each member will need to adapt. Role tasks that are no longer completed by the caregiver for other members will need to be accomplished in a new way, requiring someone else to create changes. Each time a member shifts roles, reverberations are felt by other members of the system. When other family members respond with their own changes to adapt to the initial change, inevitably their adaptations also reverberate through the system. Families can potentially experience a never-ending cycle of changes, but they rarely do, because the pressure toward predictability in systems is a powerful counterbalancing influence. In other words, family systems seek homeostasis for a very good reason—any shift in anyone's role ends up creating changes others.

Caregivers who add responsibilities for the care recipient and have fewer resources for others are likely to be missed by those family members. The reduction in the caregiver's availability to her children, husband, or siblings may leave a hole. A common scenario we encounter is the loss faced by children of a daughter caregiver of aging parents (see Figure 7.1). The daughter's nightly visits to cook for her parents and ensure that evening medications are taken appropriately have cut into family time with her own teenagers. Teens can adapt by filling the time quite easily and indeed may prefer less family time and more availability with friends. However, the loss of family time may have the cost of fewer opportunities to be guided or tracked, yielding opportunities for higher risk behaviors that could be regretted by both teens and parents.

When the caregiving role has brought growth to the caregiver, everyone around may be able to benefit. The confidence gained can position the caregiver to change careers to human services or add a volunteer role as a support group leader, for example. That same confidence may allow the caregiver to engage other family members in more productive ways rather than seeking affirmation in the face of

FIGURE 7.1

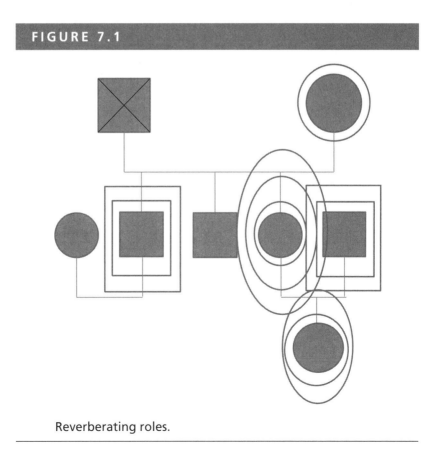

Reverberating roles.

insecurity. Widening the lens can offer the CFT therapist and client the opportunity to review gains, celebrating the benefits of expanded confidence, skills, knowledge, or abilities as they impact other relationships.

When caregiving expands role capability, the surrounding family members often can expand their own relationship with the caregiver in new ways well beyond caregiving-related topics. A caregiving son whose ability to care for his father has expanded his awareness of and comfort with his nurturant self can offer more nurturance in other relationships. Some spouses and children find themselves able to forgive past wrongs as they care for the very frail family member, thus ending a perpetual yet impossible search for approval from the older person that could never be satisfied by that person. Almost always, that perpetual search has had ramifications for other relationships as well, retaining anxiety in the hurt person that restricted the flow of love and acceptance for others. In short, caregiving for a frail person can put to rest old wrongs that obviously will never be made right by the elder who created the hurt, and that healing can also reverberate throughout the family system.

Almost always, caregiving skills and knowledge help the caregiver relate to other family members regarding other current and future elder-care scenarios. Nothing makes us more aware of our own mortality than confronting the death of a loved one. The death of the generation that precedes us is a powerful signal that we are "next up," having thus become the omega in the lineage (Hagestad, 1988). Caring for a frail elder in the months and years prior to death is our first glimpse that we not only will die but will also likely experience a period of dependency prior to death. Humans avoid discussing and preparing for the period of frailty that precedes dying as much as they avoid preparing for their own death (perhaps more). Caregiving for others teaches us about this period and what we need to do to make peace with it in our own life course.

Cultural Variations

Cultural rules about who is to provide what types of care to older family members are powerful and important to understand. CFT therapists must respect the cultural traditions behind role prescriptions for elder care, yet also must recognize the real consequences of those traditions for individuals throughout the family system. Many traditional cultures have strong prohibitions against using paid residential care settings to provide for the day-to-day needs of older family members (Pinquart & Sörensen, 2005b). "We take care of our own, in the home, where all other aspects of family life occur": This type of statement suggests a role prescription that is presumed to be shared by the cultural group.

Family norms in some cultures require that particular people fulfill particular roles in caring for aging family members. For example, some Asian cultures assign primary responsibility for parents' care to the oldest son and/or his wife (see the example in Exhibit 7.3). Options for negotiating those responsibilities may be quite limited within the cultural norms, so other family members simply have to figure out how to adapt to the changes that result from added caregiving responsibilities. On the other hand, raising the question of the impact of a particular way of providing care to older family members may invite the family to rethink the costs of traditional strategies. Second- and third-generation immigrant families may be open to considering how they are going to integrate their traditional culture with the norms of their new country. Strict adherence to old strategies may be less important to the family than loyalty to traditional values. The therapist can invite family members to consider how their dual cultural identities could free them to explore new strategies that align with closely held family values.

A very challenging aspect of acculturation is that traditional values often conflict with current lifestyle realities for recent immigrant families. Adults of the second and subsequent generations are often working hard to succeed within the values of both the traditional or home culture as well as the new culture. Long hours of paid employment to earn status in the new country, when added to other family responsibilities, may severely stress an adult child's ability to provide care for aging parents according to the rules of the original country or culture. Yet definitions of self as a good person are inevitably bound up with fulfilling long-held role expectations that may be unquestioned

EXHIBIT 7.3

Mrs. Kim

Mrs. Kim was not surprised when her son and his wife invite her to live with them because Korean cultural expectations include in-home care of older family members. She was not prepared, however, to spend so much time alone in the house. Her daughter-in-law and children seem to be always on the go, working, going to college, and socializing. Mrs. Kim becomes frightened and calls her daughter-in-law to come home, which obviously upsets her. Sometimes Mrs. Kim is afraid that her daughter-in-law is going to yell at her, but so far her son has been able to calm things down when he gets home. The couple obviously is not happy, and Mrs. Kim feels guilty about burdening them, but she is angry at her daughter-in-law for not being able to be more gracious about what is, after all, her duty. Furthermore, if her son would make his daughters stay home, they could help their mother more with the housework. Alternatively, he should just tell his wife to stay home to care for the girls and his mother. Mrs. Kim decides she shouldn't feel guilty because she is just teaching her family the Korean customs that are otherwise going to get lost.

by the first-generation immigrants who are now aging (Montgomery & Kosloski, 2011). "You are the oldest daughter, so you have to care for us; if you don't, who will?" Such statements can severely unsettle a moderately acculturated woman who expected to share parent–care responsibilities with other siblings and paid help.

Other significant cultural variations in caregiving norms, in addition to immigration and acculturation, also influence this step of balancing caregiving resources, of course. Religion and social class shape the rules for guiding family members in how to care for each other. Indeed, any social context that defines the rules for care of someone in need is a potent force in figuring out how to balance multiple responsibilities among family members. Cultural rules include dicta about who gets priority for the care and nurturance that is available within a family and who rates secondary status. In some groups, children are at the top of the list regardless, whereas other groups give priority to elderly family members.

The CFT therapist needs to listen carefully for the subtle, tacit conceptual frames that influence how caregivers balance the effects of caregiving on other roles. Regardless of culture, some caregivers have internalized frames that are unnecessarily restrictive, even within their culture, and they need to be assisted with widening the lens of possibilities for how to structure roles. For example, a daughter who perceives caring for a parent in her home as a cultural imperative may revisit the options if she notices the negative effects of her caregiving on her children. Other caregivers are in a true zero-sum game in which investment anywhere is associated with deficit somewhere else because the resources are so exceptionally limited. Without magic wands, we cannot always make resources appear. But deliberate mindful attention to the effects of caregiving on the broader network can assist caregivers in all situations in becoming conscious of what is disrupting their sense of balance among competing commitments. This first step prepares the caregiver to make conscious decisions about how to maximize the benefits of his or her care efforts within existing resources and cultural rules.

Balancing Role Commitments

The view through the wider lens may bring a sobering awareness to the caregiver that someone in his or her life is suffering because of the caregiver's commitment to care for an older family member. A caregiver may panic in the face of such a discovery because he or she feels helpless to resolve the trade-offs inherent in choosing to put the energy and resources into caregiving that seem necessary. A son who brings his father to live with his family may find that his children's lives have been altered in ways that are truly problematic. If his father is intolerant of the children's inevitable noise, messiness, or day-to-day attentional needs, the son may feel caught between his belief that his father deserves personal, in-home care from a family member and the children's misery at living under constant criticism. A husband who chose to place his wife in a nursing home on advice of their physician may be very distressed that their assets will all be used for her care, leaving nothing to help his children pay for his care or for an inheritance for their grandchildren. These examples point to the very real consequences of caregiving decisions.

The process of balancing starts with awareness of the trade-offs inherent in caregiving. Family life almost always involves trade-offs of resources such as time, energy, attention, nurturance, and finances. Humans are finite beings, so the choice to give a lot to one person means there is less for another. Few individuals or families could claim to have unlimited—or even excess—energy, time, and money. Commitment of extraordinary care to one person almost always means someone else gets less.

Although caregiving trade-offs are inevitable, the consequences should not be blatantly harmful to any family member. Therapists often hear incidental stories from caregivers about how other family members are responding to the caregiving scenario but may need to ask in a more purposive way. A review of the genogram affords the option of asking about how different members of the caregiver's family are affected by the caregiving work. The therapist might offer to facilitate a family conversation, especially with the caregiver's children, as a way of eliciting previously unspoken concerns.

Key questions to ask the caregiver include the following:

- How has your [mother/father/sister]'s role in caring for _____ changed things at home for you?
- What do you like, and not like, about how things are different?

Certainly, learning to share the limited attention and resources of a parent is a part of normal child development; similarly, caring for an older family member may open a possibility for learning and growth. Some caregivers respond to the wider lens with added guilt that their children, marriages, or other relationships are not getting as much as they had previously. The CFT therapist needs to monitor evidence of adaptation and resilience in the family members just as they track deficits in care because of diverted resources. Children can gain confidence and competence, as well as a sense of moral purpose, when they add responsibilities to the family in the face of Mom's or Dad's involvement with grandparents.

Additional resources may be needed to ensure that the full set of necessary supports for development is in place for all members of the family. If the caregiver identifies someone whose needs are not being met because of his or her investment in caregiving work, the CFT therapist can help identify ways to compensate for those strains. One option is to add paid assistance to reduce role demands at home (e.g., housecleaning services, a nanny to oversee and transport children to after-school activities). Another option is to revisit and potentially renegotiate caregiving roles, adding secondary caregivers (paid or volunteer) to reduce the load on the primary caregiver. Secondary family caregivers may also need to add resources for other family members (e.g., an aunt may agree to attend performances of a theatre student that conflict with elder-care tasks, the other parent may add cooking and clean-up to the daily routine so that family dinner experiences are maintained when the primary caregiver cannot personally deliver them as in the past). Less incidental chat time with teens may worry a caregiving daughter of aging parents who could perhaps invite a teen to join her in one task per week with the aging parents so they can talk on the way there and back.

The general principle is that caregivers need to be invited to acknowledge that caregiving commitments create reverberations throughout their family and to ensure that those are not harmful to anyone else's development. Creative problem solving can offset risks to other family members by enhancing the resources available to them, at least to the level needed to support their development. Resources may be enhanced by renegotiating the caregiver's primary roles with the care recipient, by empowering family members to grow into new roles that fill the gaps left by the caregiver, or by engaging paid or volunteer resources to fill in remaining gaps.

Anticipating the Future Without Gloom and Doom

As we complete an episode of work with a caregiving family, we pause to anticipate the future transitions in care that seem likely to occur. Without a crystal ball, we obviously cannot predict the future in detail, yet many care recipient illnesses are chronic diseases with known trajectories (Gabriel, 2011). We have two reasons for engaging clients in this anticipatory work: (a) it reinforces the notion that the caregiving journey is not static but can be expected to change significantly as the care recipients' or caregivers' needs change in the future, and (b) we want to give permission for people to return for another episode of CFT if they need to do so.

Almost all of our caregivers are working with chronic diseases that will lead in a downward trajectory toward death. Caregivers do not need to have their noses rubbed in the inevitable future. Yet they deserve to be supported in their reality rather than engaged in a delusion that if they just care well enough, the older family member will return to a previous state of well-being. In many cases, good care can indeed stabilize a person's chronic conditions, cure and/or prevent acute problems, and thus make the person better. However, *better* is a temporary status in the case of chronic disease, and family members who do not understand that fact are at risk for making poor decisions for themselves and/or the care recipient.

Anticipatory images of the future thus need to be shared gently, with respect for the fact that those images are unwelcome or at least not preferred and usually are being introduced off time for the caregivers. Neither care recipients nor caregivers really want to look very far down the road. They are trying hard to cope with the here and now and can easily become overwhelmed with what lies ahead. Thus, gentleness and a certain lightness of tone are needed to encourage the caregiver not to dwell on, or try to work out all the details of, the next stages. The future images are shared only to signal that change inevitably will come, and that change need not shock or distress the caregiver. Indeed, the inevitability of change adds to the sense that it is predictable, and thus the caregiver can anticipate finding the resources to deal with it.

Families often can benefit from doing some homework about the resources they will need in the future, so that they understand the options before the need for them becomes urgent. Many caregivers have never been inside an assisted living facility, or if they visited one, have no idea about the very wide range of options that fit within that category. Most families have no awareness of nonresidential long-term-care options such as day programs or home-based care service models. *Geriatric care management* is not exactly a commonly used term. Medical equipment showrooms display resource options that are unfamiliar to most of us. Initial conversations with agencies or residential settings can offer a relaxed exploration of service options at a time when the need for immediate decisions is not driving the process.

Specific details about the illness trajectory may be helpful to a family (Gabriel, 2011). In dementia care, for example, caregivers may find it useful to know what types of skills may be lost in the next few years so that they can monitor safety appropriately. In other words, anticipating changes from the chronic illness become the basis for anticipating changes in the caregivers' roles. Most caregivers appreciate being given what feels like a "heads up" on changes to monitor. When specific changes can be anticipated, therapists can provide resources that will

Mallory

Mallory asks her therapist to help her look ahead so that she can anticipate the key turning points in her father's care. How will she know when he is no longer safe in his environment? What signs and symptoms would indicate that he needs more assistance, like that provided in assisted living? When will she need to take over his medication administration?

become useful in the future for caregiving family members. In addition to community resources, caregivers often appreciate being able to anticipate the changes in their own roles that might add stress (see the example in Exhibit 7.4).

Some family members are interested in knowing the trajectory all the way to the end stages of the care recipient's illness. They want information about the dying process, including choices regarding hospice and palliative care. Coaching can help caregivers interview primary care physicians to obtain more specific information about the physical dying process. Unfortunately, some health care providers are uncomfortable talking about the dying process and try to redirect the family away from "worrying about that now." For some families, information is comforting, and they need to be taught how to keep asking until the physician meets their needs.

In contrast, other families cannot tolerate a conversation about any future beyond tomorrow. They want to take the changes as they come, without trying to map them out, control them, or even anticipate them. These families are highly unlikely to check out resources unless they need them now or to read about the next steps in a disease. Therapists need to measure the family's comfort with looking ahead, invite and maybe even push lightly, then back off and trust the family's wisdom in managing care in their best way possible.

Family anticipation of future transitions usually centers on safety risks. "When is it time to . . ." questions are almost always seeking signs of increased risk. Common questions address driving risk, financial management, medication management, fall risks, and meal preparation risks, which are discussed in more detail in Chapter 3 ("Structuring Care"). Less obvious questions that families may not initiate on their own are also important for therapists to consider discussing. Therapists may have to raise the topic of choosing when to advocate for more rehabilitation versus explore hospice and palliative care. When the caregiver's self-care will be so compromised that health risks increase, the therapist can anticipate the need for change in the care recipient's care structure.

Financial resources are another important topic to invite families to investigate. Multigenerational families have rules about who is allowed to know about the resources of an older adult family member. In some families, only the spouse and perhaps one adult child are expected to have that type of intimate information. Other families are happy to share at times of transition, almost as a ritual or rite accompanying significant changes. Family caregivers may appreciate coaching in how to bring up the topic of financial assets. CFT therapists can provide model language for caregivers, such as the following:

> Dad, I always want to use your resources to support you and Mother to live as independently as possible. I know nothing about how many resources you have, nor what portion is available in an emergency and which would require more planning to access. I wonder how you would feel about giving me a tutorial on how you have it all structured, where the funds are and who is a contact person I would need to use in the event you were disabled or died unexpectedly. I have no intention of trying to take over anything—I just want to be able to act in accordance with the care and planning you have used to gather these assets and to carry out your wishes with regard to any future care needs for you or Mother that you cannot handle.

Briefer model language might be, "Mom, I'm trying to find out if you qualify for some additional services or resources, so I need to know how much money you actually have in the bank. By the way, is anyone but you a signer on any of those accounts?"

Aging family members tend to have a certain pride in independence that must be respected even in the face of poverty or extreme frailty. As the birth cohort who experienced the Great Depression firsthand, those ages 80 to 100+ years are likely to have worked hard to protect others from being burdened financially. Regardless of the size of the nest egg, there is a certain pride in saving and self-management of finance. Older family members tend to prefer to retain privacy around the amount of their assets, which must be respected. However, they can also be reminded of the very good reasons for sharing some information at least, so that others are less burdened in the event of an emergency.

Termination of an Episode of CFT Work

When the caregiver roles are stable and the needs of care recipient and caregiver are met, therapy can be ended, at least for now. CFT is intended to be time limited, with the purpose of helping the family obtain stability in a caregiving structure that meets the needs of both caregiver and care recipient without having a negative impact on other family members or the system's functioning. We conceptualize the work as occurring in episodes, with a chunk devoted to stabilizing the family caregiving situation around the current care needs. Future changes may or may not send the family back for another episode of work. We have many families that return every 2 to 3 years for a few sessions, after which we hear nothing until the care needs unsettle the family again. Other families do one episode of work in CFT and figure out how to respond to future shifts in care on their own.

The CFT therapist and client work together to determine when the CFT work is done. Often the demands of caregiving are sufficient that an extra appointment for therapy may actually be a burden. Clients may be vigilant for the earliest opportunity to reduce that added burden or may be reluctant to let go of a true source of support for their remarkable work. The therapist needs to play a role in helping the client revisit the problem(s) that brought them in initially and to review what is known about the care recipient's needs, the adequacy and stability of care structures, and the well-being of the main caregivers. The process of widening the lens also affords the therapist an opportunity to raise questions about what appear to be logical or inevitable challenges within the family, given the structures of care and the dynamics of the family. Certainly, caregivers sometimes end an episode of CFT before the therapist believes the family is stabilized in its caregiving work. Termination of therapy before the work appears to be done is not uncommon, and therapists must learn to observe, document their concerns, and at some level hope or trust that the family knows how to proceed from here without crisis. Obviously, hope and trust are not always realistic, and the CFT therapist, like all other therapists, learns to let go of the client who appears headed in the wrong direction when he or she insists on going down that path.

The opposite problem also arises in CFT occasionally: A caregiving family may not ever seem to improve in functioning. In some cases, the therapist needs to ratchet up the intensity of the family-level intervention. For example, more members of the family may need to be engaged in the room so the therapist can facilitate conversations that the caregiver client may not have been able to handle independently. In other cases, the therapist needs to rethink the functioning of the caregivers in the family, looking for possible longer term personality disorders or significant mental health dysfunction. Personality disorders render people less flexible to shift focus or strategy without very significant support. CFT strategies are focused on changes in relationship structures that empower and enable people to change, but personality disorders make those changes very difficult to understand or implement. Severe thought disorders (e.g., schizophrenia), depression, or substance abuse might also impede clients from collaborating on new strategies. When CFT strategies are not proceeding toward change, or are not achieving new stable structures, therapists are encouraged to review the need for individual or family psychotherapy that is targeted less at shifts in caregiving than at treatment of, or intervention with, the functioning of the caregivers.

As an episode of CFT is completed, we encourage a careful process of termination that engages the therapist and client in a review of the work accomplished, claiming the gains that have been made and celebrating growth. Termination always involves noting disappointments about therapy as well, unrealized hopes for change that perhaps were not realistic or at least were not yet accomplished. The care taken in termination is foundational to the invitation to return for another episode when the care structures and strategies no longer work for the family.

Key questions to ask the caregiver include the following:

- How have your beliefs about the care recipient's situation changed since you started coming here? What did you believe when you arrived? What do you believe now?
- What changes did you make in your own caregiving role during therapy?
- What changes did others make in their caregiving roles, and how were those changes created?
- Who made them? How were you involved? What is their impact on you?
- How are you caring for yourself now? What have you learned about maintaining good self-care?
- What are you anticipating in the future care picture?

The therapist usually leads the client through a review of the therapeutic relationship as well as the therapy process. The relationship conversation allows the client to reflect on how he or she connected with the therapist as a person, as well as in the therapist role. The reflection also includes a review of how the relationship was structured. Because CFT often engages the primary therapist in drawing in other family members, some reflection about that process is useful because it names the processes that can be used in the future. Caregivers who brought other family members into secondary caregiving roles to build support will likely need to ask them to change their forms of assistance as the care recipient's needs change. The strategies that worked during this episode of therapy may also work in the future, so helping the client label exactly what happened should give guidance to the client for the future. Although CFT is not deep intrapsychically oriented therapy, termination still offers an opportunity for the client to consolidate a model for help seeking that is positive, proactive, and self-aware.

Key questions to ask the caregiver include the following:

- What did we do together to make this a safe place to talk about these difficult family matters?
- What did I do in the therapy that was particularly useful to you? Not useful?
- When we decided to include your family members, what process did we use that you think might be useful to you in the future?

Death of a Care Recipient

Care recipients are almost always quite ill or disabled and so are at high risk of dying during therapy. CFT therapists can sometimes anticipate a pending death, and indeed part of the work with the caregiver may be focused on preparations for dying. However, unanticipated deaths also occur, launching the caregiver and therapist into a different type of work quite unexpectedly. Postdeath work is very much a part of CFT, with a focus on transitioning the caregiver out of the role by ending it well. Certainly, some caregiving clients call to report that the care recipient has died, with the intent of therapy ending at that point. We suggest that CFT therapists strongly encourage the caregiving client to come in for at least a final session in order to process through the termination work described previously. The weeks immediately following the death may not be a great time to do that final session because the work of planning a memorial, dealing with the personal items of the deceased, and handling the emotional load of grief may be overwhelming. For some caregivers, the ideal time frame is 1 to 2 months later, at which point the caregiver can report on the postdeath activities and reactions and tie together the CFT work (see the example in Exhibit 7.5).

EXHIBIT 7.5

Lynn

Lynn called to report to her CFT therapist that her mother had died unexpectedly last night. She was obviously crying when she left the voice message, and she indicated that she was grateful for the help received and would not be returning now that she was no longer a caregiver. The CFT therapist returned the call, offering condolences along with a session to process the death. Lynn returned the call to say that she was really too busy to have a session right now and indeed was grieving with strong supports around her. Lynn accepted the therapist's offer to call again in about a month to see about setting up a final session during which they could process all that was happening around the time of the death.

Life after caregiving can be a stressful transition for a family member and may prompt reentry into therapy for assistance with the post-caregiving transition. The role of caregiver is often one that the family member has adopted and owned for a long time such that the death of the care recipient propels the caregiver into grief for both the loved one and the caregiving role. In addition to the more obvious need for the therapist to address grief and bereavement for the loss of the care recipient, the caregiving therapist needs to address the loss of the caregiving role. Most caregivers have devoted a significant amount of time and energy to their loved ones, often having had daily, weekly, or monthly routines that were followed. After the care recipient's death, the family member may be at a loss for how to spend the time that is now solely his or her own. Therapists should be aware of any feelings of anger, guilt, or hopelessness that may appear during this transition out of the caregiving role and help the family member in addressing them.

Conclusion

As the family adjusts to its caregiving role structures and strategies, the therapist invites the clients to widen the lens, looking at the effects of the current caregiving plan on the well-being of the wider family system and its members. The goal of most families is, at a minimum, to harm no member, and thus the widening-the-lens checkup is welcomed by families who seek to ensure that all members can develop and function effectively. CFT clients are also invited to anticipate future transitions in caregiving. When the caregiving structures are stable and functioning reasonably well, CFT attempts to end each episode with a termination process that includes review of the therapy process, relationship, and options for accessing help in the future. The death of the care recipient during CFT engages therapists and clients in looking beyond caregiving to yet another family structure transition.

Case Studies 8

Two cases are presented in this chapter to illustrate the unfolding intervention processes of caregiver family therapy (CFT). Both cases are an amalgam of real families with whom we have worked. Many details have been changed to help us both mask the identities of the family and illustrate the CFT processes more clearly.

Linda

Linda is caring for her mother, Mrs. Johnson, from a considerable distance. She has three siblings who are concerned but less involved than she is. Mrs. Johnson is showing signs of cognitive impairment that had worried Linda for quite a while before she initiated CFT. This case illustrates some of the dynamics experienced by siblings who care for a parent from a long distance away. This European American family

DOI: 10.1037/13943-008
Caregiver Family Therapy: Empowering Families to Meet the Challenges of Aging,
by S. H. Qualls and A. A. Williams

places strong value on individual development, boundaries, and maximizing autonomy.

ENTERING CFT (CHAPTER 1)

Linda was one of the lucky ones—she became a caregiver with an abundance of personal and professional resources. Yet despite an advanced degree and successful career as an educator, significant financial resources, and siblings who were willing to help her, Linda was distressed by her mother's decline and her own confusion about how to handle it. Mrs. Johnson was a highly educated person living alone in the same house where she and her now-deceased husband had lived for decades in a small university town. Until last year, she had maintained a full social life, volunteer activities, and an impressive physical exercise regimen for a woman in her 80s. During Linda's recent visits, she noticed that her mother seemed less engaged with friends than she had been throughout her life. Mrs. Johnson had few events listed on her calendar and was not worried about it. She also was uninterested in cooking or even going out to eat. Her biggest worry was that Linda was there to make her move, and she wanted desperately to stay where she was. Most concerning were the frequent repeated questions and moments of obvious forgetting of what happened only hours ago.

While visiting her mother, Linda called the local Area Agency on Aging for a referral to a case manager or therapist who could help her figure out whether she should be worried and, if so, what to do. She was referred to a clinical geropsychologist, who, along with social work and case manager colleagues in her office, offered caregiver interventions for families. Linda gratefully took her first appointment.

NAMING THE PROBLEM (CHAPTER 2)

Linda realized that her three brothers were devoted to their mother but from a distance, so they all had different impressions of how Mother was doing. She worried about what would happen when her mother needed more care. Would the boys get involved? Would they ever be able to be on the same page about her care? Would her sister-in-law, who lives nearest to mother, be willing to step in to help, given that Mother had been so critical of her through the years?

The CFT therapist gathered detailed information about Linda's observations, along with some history on Mrs. Johnson and the family. She guided Linda to schedule a physical examination with Mrs. Johnson and a neuropsychological evaluation during Linda's next visit. The physical exam showed evidence that Mrs. Johnson's long-term thyroid medication dosages needed to be increased and a potassium supplement was needed.

The physician recommended waiting until hormone and electrolyte levels were within normal range before proceeding with the neuropsychological exam because deficiencies in either could cause cognitive problems. So Linda postponed all other evaluations for 2 months. After 2 months had passed, Linda visited her mother again, and at that time blood levels were measured and showed that she was now at normal levels. Unfortunately, Linda saw the same memory problems and social withdrawal that had become characteristic of her mother's behavior in the past year or two. She was advised to proceed with the neuropsychological evaluation.

Mrs. Johnson was quite resistant to being tested, claiming she "was not crazy" and that besides, everyone knew that "those stupid standardized tests aren't relevant to everyday life." She was angry at Linda for suggesting the evaluation and flatly refused to schedule it. Linda met with the CFT therapist for help. She was invited to think about how she would respond if the recommended tests were blood tests that her mother was refusing. Linda was a bit startled by the question and realized that she would have no difficulty telling her mother quite simply, "We are doing this" for tests of physical functioning. She applied that approach to this situation and proceeded to schedule the test; she simply announced to her mother that these tests were "important to the doctor so we should try them. No harm done in doing them because you might turn out to be just fine." Mrs. Johnson grumbled but quit arguing.

Linda accompanied her mother to the neuropsychological evaluation, where Linda was interviewed about her behavioral observations. She was grateful because she feared her mother would simply say nothing was wrong. Linda was dismayed to learn that she would have to return in 2 weeks to hear the results of the test, but she agreed to schedule another visit. This would make four flights to be with her mother in 3 months—quite a costly enterprise. She believed she was the best person to guide her mother through the evaluation process, though, because her brothers were not likely to insist on proceeding despite her mother's protests. She wondered how many more flights lay ahead this year.

When the neuropsychologist met with Mrs. Johnson and Linda together to go over the results of the test, he described several areas of cognitive function in which Mrs. Johnson was performing quite normally and noted some areas of mild or moderate impairment in memory and executive functioning. He suggested that it was too early to offer a specific diagnosis but that the pattern of difficulties looked like it was more than just normal aging, with a good possibility of being caused by tiny strokes. He suggested retesting her in another 6 months to see if he could contribute to a diagnosis that he suspected would be vascular dementia.

He also recommended follow-up with Mrs. Johnson's primary care provider for an evaluation that included brain imaging. Mrs. Johnson heard the results without any apparent concern, agreeing that sometimes she has trouble with those skills but "nothing that affects my everyday life." She was relieved that "at least it wasn't Alzheimer's disease!" Having no further questions, Mrs. Johnson was quite content to wait for Linda, who wanted some private time with the doctor.

Following are Linda's key questions for the doctor:

- How did he reach his conclusions?
- What exactly is vascular dementia, and how do you treat it?
- What is the trajectory ahead?
- Is she in danger living alone? And if not yet, how will they know when?
- Is it OK for her to drive?

Linda left the feedback session with a heavy heart and struggled to find lighter topics to discuss with her mother on the ride home. Mrs. Johnson again stated her relief that she did not have Alzheimer's disease and that Linda could relax now that everything was just fine. She made it clear she did not want to talk any more about the "work of that fine young man."

Linda met with her CFT therapist to figure out what to do next. The neuropsychologist had not been very specific in his answers to Linda's questions. He kept emphasizing that retesting needed to be done in 6 months to allow him to be more definitive. Meanwhile, Linda wanted some guidance. Most immediately, how and what should she tell her brothers? How should she plan for her own future? Flying back and forth from home to her mother's every month was just not feasible.

Linda decided to share the report with her brothers and added a cover letter explaining what she understood the report to mean. The CFT therapist reviewed the cover letter, corrected a few details, and helped Linda think through what she wanted to ask of her brothers. She also guided Linda to ask her mother for permission to share the report. The therapist explained that although Linda saw evidence that her mother was not understanding everything about her health, her mother was in fact her own legal decision maker, so Linda had no right to share information without her permission. Mrs. Johnson was unconcerned about sharing the report ("It doesn't really say anything anyway"). Linda concluded her cover letter by asking her brothers to come together on a conference phone call facilitated by the therapist to go over these results. To her surprise, they all agreed.

The therapist started the call by asking each person to share his or her current concerns about their mother, starting with Linda, who had initiated these evaluations. Each of the three brothers had a different take on their mother, with two stating emphatically that this was all a lot of fuss about nothing. One brother was more aligned with Linda in his observations, but he noted that his wife was the one who seemed more worried about what it all meant. The therapist then asked their permission to review the written report in some detail. She discussed the findings in each cognitive domain, offering suggestions about how Mrs. Johnson's performance would affect daily life. They discussed together the practical problems that currently existed and those that were likely to emerge next. The therapist offered to summarize that discussion on paper, along with some suggestions for strategies to maximize Mrs. Johnson's independence while ensuring her safety.

STRUCTURING CARE (CHAPTER 3)

High on the list of practical problems Linda wanted to address was her mother's social withdrawal. Mrs. Johnson seemed to be sitting in her house for days at a time without seeing anyone. Next in priority was Linda's concern about how to handle Mrs. Johnson's bills, which didn't seem to be paid in a timely way. The therapist asked her about Mrs. Johnson's medication schedule and whether Linda thought her mother was taking medications regularly. Linda was surprised because she really hadn't thought about that. On checking, she found that her mother clearly was not taking all of her medications because Mrs. Johnson could not open some of the pill bottles! Finally, Linda wondered whether she should be worried about her mother's driving. Mrs. Johnson only went to church on Sunday and to the grocery store once a week, but losing her car would be devastating to her. Furthermore, she was unlikely to agree to give up the car without a major fight, and Linda was pretty sure her brothers would not back her up on that. The neuropsychologist had indicated that Mrs. Johnson's level of cognitive function suggested increased risk but was too high for anyone to state definitively that she lacked the capacity to drive. To begin the problem-solving process from a positive orientation, the CFT therapist began the intervention by reassuring Linda that the problems with which she was wrestling were indeed solvable.

The therapist helped Linda identify intervention options that she had not known existed. Using the problem-solving method, they evaluated the pros and cons of various options for addressing these three problems. All three problems shared an underlying difficulty with remembering to do something in a timely way. Ultimately, Linda chose to buy her mother a large calendar that could sit on the coffee table in the living room beside her portable phone. Mrs. Johnson was grateful for the larger print version and agreed that Linda could put some appointments on there for her ("But I don't really need it"). A pen and bright pink marker were attached to the calendar with a string, so Mrs. Johnson could easily add events to the calendar and could use the pink marker each night to cross off that day. This seemed to help her track what day it was more easily and check each morning for that day's activities.

To prompt more social connections, the therapist encouraged Linda to put on the calendar the regular events that Mrs. Johnson used to do (and still enjoyed) so she could be prompted to attend them without having to recall the list on her own. Linda marked the calendar each week with the Tuesday morning Bible study at church and the Thursday afternoon bridge party. She was disappointed that Mrs. Johnson often still did not go ("I just didn't get around in time"), but Linda could at least point her mother to her calendar when they spoke on the phone. Linda realized her mother was sometimes confused about what day it was, and Mrs. Johnson became quite defensive if asked something she did not know.

Linda marked the calendar with the due dates of specific bills. She realized, however, that Mrs. Johnson was unlikely to keep her bills organized and easily identifiable. They created a special box to keep bills in, separate from other mail. After a few months, however, Linda realized that her mother could not sort the mail consistently and thus the bill box was not working. She offered to be her mother's secretary for "some of this complicated stuff, just for a while, to see if you like not having to deal with it," which Mrs. Johnson accepted with grumbles about "people taking over my life." Linda and Mrs. Johnson visited the bank together to set up online bill payment, and Linda arranged for bills to be sent to her electronically. Although it was complicated to get it all transitioned to her, Linda found the system easy to use, and her mother never asked about it again. Years later, Linda was grateful to have had access to see payments online because she was able to identify quickly a scam investment her mother made.

Linda sympathized with her mother's difficulties opening medication bottles and suggested that they use a medication reminder box with small compartments for morning, noon, and evening medications. Although she thought her mother could use this system to take pills appropriately, Linda was certain her mother could not fill the medication box accurately. Linda found a home health agency that would send a nurse weekly to refill the medication box. Mrs. Johnson doubted she could afford that level of help, but Linda assured her that Linda would pay for it because this was for Linda's peace of mind. The first nurse was "totally unacceptable" to Mrs. Johnson, who summarily fired her. Linda asked the agency to try again and insisted that her mother also try again because "this is really important to me." After a few visits, Mrs. Johnson began to look forward to the new nurse's visits and was pleasantly surprised when the nurse offered to add a quick check of blood pressure and pulse oxygen to her visit. (Mrs. Johnson thought she was getting a free service from this nice lady, so it was a really good deal!) Linda hadn't realized how comforting it would be to have someone in her mother's house every week to check that everything was OK. Over time, Linda came to believe that she was actually quite good at working through problems related to her mother's care needs.

ROLE STRUCTURES: CHALLENGES AND INTERVENTIONS (CHAPTER 4)

The role structure problems in Linda's and Mrs. Johnson's families unfolded around three dynamics: (a) Linda and her brothers viewed their mother's functional status and needs differently, so they were not positioned to agree on what family roles were needed to support her; (b) communications about roles were unfolding in patterns congruent with long-term dynamics; and (c) secondary caregiving roles were not well-defined, and role assignments were ambiguous for them.

Mrs. Johnson's four children were scattered across the United States, with active families of their own. Furthermore, all of them had learned to keep their distance because of her acidic, intrusive communication style. Now, they all agreed that Mom was "slipping" but disagreed about how much and what it meant. Even the neuropsychological evaluation did not satisfy two of the sons that something was really wrong because no diagnosis was given. Linda's work with Mom was appreciated but maybe a bit overboard in their eyes. Sending a nurse in once a week seemed like too much for a woman who was so proud and independent.

The CFT therapist worked with Linda to create her family genogram (see Figure 8.1). Linda's family contained three generations, with vertical ties and horizontal structural ties created by marital and other partnerships and by childbearing. Linda was the only daughter, although her generation also contained two women who were daughters-in-law. The bonds and conflicts were depicted with connector lines that reflected relationship dynamics—straight lines were bonds and crinkled lines were conflicts, with more lines reflecting greater strength.

After creating and contemplating the genogram, Linda became frustrated that she was doing all of this work without any help from her brothers. They needed to be more involved, but how and when? And how could she navigate the complex sibling relationships without adding stress to her life? She felt so angry after talking on the phone with them because they obviously did not believe she needed to be doing what she was doing for their mother. Yet their mother was going to need all of them during this journey, even the son she had cut off when he came out as gay. How were they ever going to work together if they couldn't get on the same page? Why didn't they trust her?

FIGURE 8.1

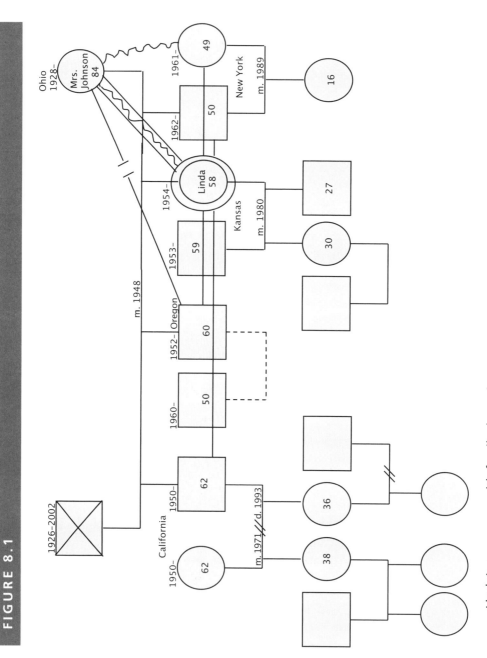

Linda's genogram with family dynamics.

Linda worked with the CFT therapist to become specific about what she wanted her brothers to do. Together they formed a plan. She was going to ask her oldest and youngest brothers to either schedule a trip to check on Mrs. Johnson or invite her to visit them during the next 6 months. She was going to leave them responsible for making the arrangements despite the temptation to help prepare. Linda was apprehensive that her mother would not be able to pack appropriately, or manage the airports, but she agreed to simply suggest to her brothers that they arrange for wheelchair transport for her and let them take it from there.

Both sons invited Mrs. Johnson for a visit, which delighted but overwhelmed her. She agreed to visit the son in California but refused to schedule other travel. Mrs. Johnson missed the flight to California the first time. She had not arranged for a taxi to take her to the airport and got quite distressed when no one arrived to pick her up. She called Linda quite upset, and Linda asked her to call the brother in California to let him know what happened. He was upset and frustrated with his mother but assured her that they would reschedule. The next time, he arranged the taxi and other details of travel. Mrs. Johnson arrived in California with an odd assortment of clothing that included no pants or skirts, so they had to purchase several new outfits for her. She looked worried and disheveled during much of the trip. She also refused to go to restaurants or other outings with his family.

The experience was eye-opening for all of the children. After the first trip, the youngest brother and his wife decided to visit her rather than arrange for her to travel. Their visit also surprised them. Mrs. Johnson had an odd assortment of food in the house and seemed to rely solely on microwaveable meals. She had no interest in cooking and was not managing to keep the house very clean. They left upset, with a sense that something had to be done.

Linda asked the CFT therapist to convene another conference call for the siblings. After a brief update, the therapist used a values clarification exercise: What was most important to them about their mother's life from now until the day she dies? Each of them insisted that they wanted her to be as happy as possible, but all felt helpless to make that happen. She had never been a particularly happy woman. All also noted in their own words that they hoped she could stay in her own home as long as possible and yet expressed fear that she was not very safe currently. The therapist helped the four siblings create a plan for adding paid caregiving support for Mrs. Johnson in her home to support basic care: hygiene, nutrition, hydration, and some human contact. Linda agreed to hire a care manager to oversee the services needed, and the sons agreed to divide the costs of paid staff and Linda's travel with her. All four discussed what type of communication they wanted with

Mrs. Johnson during her final years, a conversation that was hardest for her second son, whom she had cut off when she learned that he was gay. He expressed his deep desire to talk with her and attempt a final peace but also was cautious about upsetting her and himself. He agreed to think further about how he wanted to handle this and to consider sending her a card or brief note as a way to test her current reaction to him. Linda suggested he time the arrival of his note with her next visit so she could observe their mother's reaction and perhaps even talk with her about that relationship.

ROLE REVERBERATIONS (CHAPTER 5)

Linda found the frequent travel to be physically taxing and disruptive to her marriage. Although he had been remarkably supportive of her travel, Linda's husband had grown increasingly impatient with her emotional roller coasters. He wanted her brothers to take more responsibility and pushed Linda to make them do more of the travel. Linda cut back on almost all of her volunteer roles and found that although she didn't miss the work, she really missed the regular contact with her friends who volunteered with her.

Linda's nurse practitioner referred her to a psychotherapist for help managing the stress that was showing up as elevated blood pressure and weight gain. The psychotherapist consulted with the CFT therapist and chose to work with Linda on balancing the roles in her life with her caregiving role. Linda reestablished herself in one volunteer role that could be flexible around her travel and set social visits twice a week with friends she was missing. Linda decided not to use her husband as the sounding board for her family frustrations, and he dropped some of his grumpiness about her family. They established a date night again, a practice they used to do when the kids were little. They agreed not to talk about her family problems or his work on date night and found that they both really had fun playing together again. Linda began to feel less pulled in a thousand directions.

SELF-CARE (CHAPTER 6)

Linda recognized that for the past year she had felt tense most of the time and had been increasingly short with her husband and family. The therapist's review of Linda's self-care strategies identified that she began to worry about her mother in the evening and that worry was disrupting her sleep. They strategized a new evening routine that included good sleep hygiene behaviors. Each evening she chose one of her favorite distracters (hot tea and a movie, wine and a talk with a friend, a good book) and enjoyed it until she was genuinely sleepy.

Linda also identified exercise that she could enjoy three to four times each week. Walking was her favorite, so the therapist encouraged her to invite a friend to be a walking buddy. She was delighted when her neighbor agreed. Within a few weeks, they had established a routine that they then expanded to include walking to the gym, lifting weights, drinking juice, and walking home.

Linda still struggled with her worry and was encouraged to journal her fears and hopes for her mother. She had forgotten what a great release it was to put fears on paper and was able to cut short her long sessions of rumination with a solid journaling session followed by a favorite activity.

The added exercise and improved sleep reduced Linda's overall tension level, making it easier for her to manage her worry. Gradually, she was able to maintain a sense of healthy life at home in between visits to her mother. The care manager overseeing her mother's needs learned to give Linda solutions along with any problems she brings up, so Linda felt less alone in problem solving for her mother's care. With her renewed social network, Linda had begun to enjoy life again, not feeling quite so intensively burdened by her mother's declining health. When Mrs. Johnson fell and broke a hip, the care manager helped Linda and her brothers think through alternatives for rehabilitation and supports for Mrs. Johnson during her recovery. When it became obvious that Mrs. Johnson couldn't return home safely, all agreed that Linda and one brother would choose an assisted living residence during a joint visit.

WIDENING THE LENS AND ANTICIPATING THE FUTURE (CHAPTER 7)

During the roller coaster ride of caring for her mother, Linda had not attended very closely to her children. Thankfully, both were grown. Linda was encouraged by her therapist to schedule a long conversation as a check-in with each of her children to see how they were faring in light of less contact with their mother. She was surprised to learn that her daughter had been trying to get pregnant and that her son feared for his job because of the downturn in the economy. Neither had mentioned these previously, and Linda felt sad that she had been unavailable to support them. Lunch in a fancy restaurant with her daughter included lots of laughter and a sense of reconnecting around the joys and hopes for pregnancy. Her daughter invited Linda to attend the next fertility appointment with her, a moment of trust Linda deeply appreciated. Linda and her husband traveled to visit their son so he could feel the shared support from both of them during this stressful time. He confessed his fears of being a failure so early in his career, and they were able to help him think differently about the realities of job losses during a fragile economy. Linda realized that both of them were affected also by their grandmother's decline. Although neither had felt exceptionally close to Mrs. Johnson, both recognized that Grandma was no longer "herself" and that the grandchildren were facing mortality as a reality within their family. Both seemed to appreciate hearing Linda's account of their grandmother's difficulties. They wanted to be supportive but were not sure how to do that best. Linda suggested asking the care manager for ideas and for assistance in setting up a video conference with each of them during one of her visits with Mrs. Johnson.

Lupé and Julio

Lupé is caring for her husband, Julio, whose physical impairments are changing their lifestyle. The challenges of caregiving within a marital couple are illustrated in this case, as are some important influences of cultural variations on caregiving patterns (the couple is Mexican American). Living within a familistic culture, this couple is embedded in a system of strong family ties.

ENTERING CFT (CHAPTER 1)

Lupé and Julio recently retired and were just beginning to enjoy a more relaxed routine than when Julio was working as a high school teacher and Lupé as a librarian. They were looking forward to traveling the country in their newly purchased motor home. However, Julio had begun complaining that he did not have the energy that he once had. At a recent medical appointment, his primary care provider (PCP) diagnosed Julio with Type 2 diabetes and cardiovascular disease. The PCP also stated that Julio was at risk for cancer and chronic obstructive pulmonary disease (COPD), especially if he did not stop smoking. Lupé began to feel stress, worry, and fear about the future, concerns that previously never crossed her mind. After briefly mentioning this stress to a doctor at one of these appointments, Lupé learned of a therapist at the health care clinic who offered CFT; she made an appointment with the CFT therapist.

NAMING THE PROBLEM (CHAPTER 2)

The CFT therapist encouraged Lupé to speak with Julio's PCP about further tests. The PCP indicated that Julio needed to be assessed for COPD with a spirometry test, cancer with a chest x-ray, and his risk of having an aortic aneurism using an ultrasound. Lupé began to fear the worst but agreed that it would be best to have the information from the tests in order to obtain a clearer picture of Julio's health conditions and to avoid misunderstandings about his level of care needs. Lupé then began taking her husband to appointment after appointment for health assessments and to see her and Julio's future a little more clearly. After completing a full family history, cholesterol and blood pressure checks, and an assessment of Julio's other risk factors, Lupé was extremely thankful that her husband currently had no signs of cancer. His PCP told Lupé and Julio that he would be watching him for symptoms of COPD.

Although Lupé was disappointed that she and Julio would be unable to make their usual cross-country trip to see their oldest son that year, she began to adjust to the lifestyle changes being recommended by Julio's doctors and agreed that making a long trip would be stressful to them both. Julio now had to maintain a strict new diet; his PCP encouraged Julio to walk for exercise and strongly recommended that he stop smoking. Julio was interested in making these changes; however, he struggled on a day-to-day basis with implementing (and sticking to) these adjustments. He and Lupé both worried because if he was unable to make these lifestyle changes, he might have to take medications, and his health would only get worse and worse.

Six months after Julio received diagnoses of Type 2 diabetes and cardiovascular disease, his PCP also told Lupé and Julio that he had COPD. Julio had been noticing shortness of breath, lethargy, and an inability to focus, all of which were related to poor blood oxygen saturation levels. Lupé wondered what this would mean for her and her husband in the upcoming months and years. Julio's PCP told him that he would likely be on oxygen for the rest of his life.

Julio also mentioned that several times over the past few months he had become disoriented while driving, and the PCP indicated that he needed a driving assessment to determine whether he was safe driving with his current conditions. Unfortunately, the driving assessment indicated that Julio was at risk of getting into an accident because of his deteriorating vision, along with low oxygen levels, which can cause sleepiness and poor attention to details in the environment that are important to notice while driving.

STRUCTURING CARE (CHAPTER 3)

Lupé worked with her CFT therapist and decided that the primary problem she needed to address with Julio was his driving. She had never been the one to drive the two of them, and she felt awkward mentioning that a change was needed. Lupé's therapist facilitated the rational problem-solving process with Lupé, and she decided that she would talk with Julio's PCP and ask whether she could tell Julio that he was becoming unsafe to drive. Lupé followed through with the steps she had outlined in therapy by talking with Julio's PCP, and Julio, though he was unhappy about the news that he should no longer be driving, followed his PCP's recommendations and gave his keys to Lupé. He decided it was better for her to be the driver than to rely on their children or the senior agency van.

ROLE STRUCTURING (CHAPTER 4)

Lupé's therapist drew a genogram of her family to show Lupé the current caregiving structure within her family (see Figure 8.2). Lupé and Julio have four adult children who live nearby and one adult son who lives in another state. All of their children are married, and their four oldest children have children of their own. Lupé and Julio have always been very happy and thankful to have close relationships with their sons and daughters. Lupé noticed that she was the only person in her family providing care to Julio, but she was unsure how to let go of pieces of her role as the primary caregiver.

When Lupé and Julio and their family gathered for the holidays this year, several of their children were surprised to notice that the couple seemed frailer than they had in the past. During their monthly visits to their parents' house, the children had not noticed the gradual changes in their parents. When their parents were in their own home, it was harder to notice changes in their functioning, but when they visited their daughter's house and Julio had to contend with climbing stairs, Julio's weakness was more apparent, and Lupé appeared more tired than usual. The children reasoned that in their own home, Lupé and Julio had an easier time masking the true level of difficulties they were experiencing. They noticed very clearly for the first time at Thanksgiving that Lupé's role demands were simply more than she could manage alone, and the children decided to each increase their support to their parents. Lupé's oldest daughter, Maria, talked with her brothers and sisters, and they all agreed to pitch in and do more to help. When Maria approached Lupé and told her what she and her other brothers and sisters wanted to do, Lupé said that she could not accept their help. She said that she did not want to disrupt their busy lives and that she was managing well enough.

Upset about her children's observations regarding her and Julio's declining health, Lupé made another appointment with the CFT therapist to discuss the matter. The CFT therapist worked with Lupé and encouraged her to accept help from her children. The nearby adult family members were invited to a CFT session, where they worked with

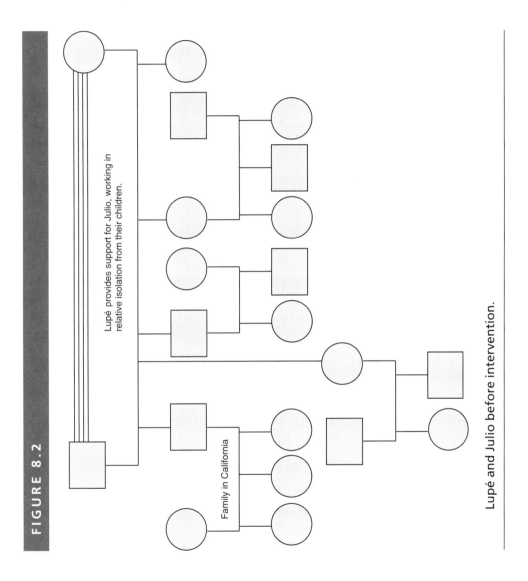

FIGURE 8.2

Lupé provides support for Julio, working in relative isolation from their children.

Family in California

Lupé and Julio before intervention.

Lupé, Julio, and the therapist to create a schedule that involved having someone visit Lupé and Julio on a daily basis, assisting with grocery shopping and meal preparation several times a week, and doing home repairs as needed. Because the couple had a large family, the burden was not too great on any family member, and Lupé said that although she had worried about being a burden at first, she was actually relieved to have so much assistance. She also said that she preferred having family members coming in to the home to asking strangers to help with Julio's needs.

During their next therapy session, the therapist drew an updated version of Lupé's family genogram (see Figure 8.3). The therapist complimented Lupé on the changes she and her family had made to distribute care for Julio more equally among the family members and emphasized to Lupé that her sons, daughters, and grandchildren could be great supports for her and Julio in the future.

ROLE REVERBERATIONS (CHAPTER 5)

Lupé and Julio settled into a routine in which Lupé took over driving, and she became comfortable with her new role as his health care manager, taking him to appointments, following diet regimens, and monitoring his oxygen levels. Yet Lupé's daughter, Maria, noticed her mother seemed strained during their last several visits. Maria asked her mother on several occasions whether she was still attending church and whether she had spent any time with her friends, and Lupé always responded no. Lupé certainly missed these activities, but she also felt that it was all she could do to maintain her energy while fulfilling all of her current responsibilities caring for Julio. Lupé brought up Maria's concerns the next time she saw her therapist and stated that she was not sure how to manage caregiving while also attempting to get back to her old routines at church. The therapist asked Lupé whether Maria might be an available resource to help her, especially given that Maria had brought up her concerns that Lupé was no longer involved in many of the activities she once enjoyed.

Lupé talked with Maria and indicated that she did not feel comfortable leaving Julio home alone, even for short periods of time. Maria emphasized to her mother that Julio's PCP had said he would be fine for short periods of time at home alone, but Lupé was unrelenting in her fear of leaving him. Maria offered to have Julio over to her home for breakfast on Sunday mornings as a way of spending time with her father and also encouraging her mother to go back to her Sunday church services. Lupé agreed to give this a try, even though she was skeptical about whether Julio would agree to go to Maria's every week. Lupé was surprised how much Julio seemed to enjoy the time with Maria and realized it was good for both of them to have some time apart.

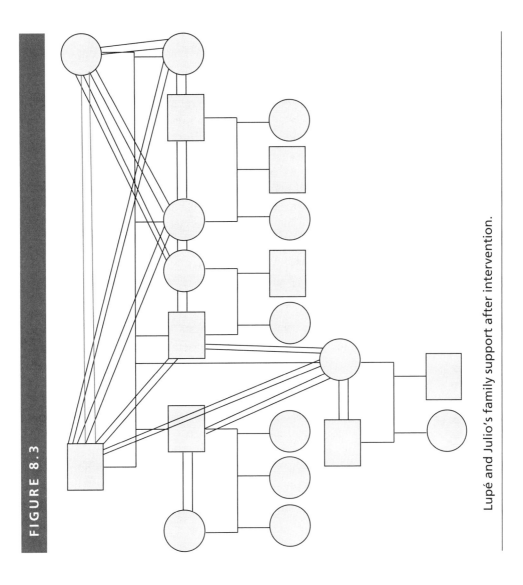

FIGURE 8.3

Lupé and Julio's family support after intervention.

SELF-CARE (CHAPTER 6)

Lupé had been caring for her husband for several months when she came to therapy one day and said that she felt more comfortable in her current roles and was beginning to adjust to her husband's illness. At the same time, however, she said that she was beginning to worry about her own health because she had not been able to maintain an exercise routine while caring for Julio. The CFT therapist helped Lupé clarify her values, and Lupé decided that exercising was absolutely a priority, and she wanted to begin as soon as she could.

The CFT therapist worked with Lupé to apply problem-solving techniques. Lupé came up with several strategies for integrating exercise back into her weekly routine. She called a neighbor and asked whether the neighbor would be willing to visit with Julio in the afternoons for about 15 minutes a day so that Lupé could walk around the block. She also invited Maria to go to the YMCA with her once a week, and Maria agreed. Lupé also asked Maria to bring her children over on Saturdays every other weekend because she found that caring for their grandchildren kept her and Julio energized and active.

WIDENING THE LENS AND ANTICIPATING THE FUTURE (CHAPTER 7)

Lupé had a final session with her CFT therapist, at which time she discussed her views of the future. Lupé said that she felt her life was stable caring for Julio, and she was pleased with her children's increased involvement in their lives. Lupé knew that she might be caring for Julio for several years, and she anticipated when changes might come in the future and what they might look like.

During this final CFT session, Lupé also thought about whether she and Julio should consider moving into a smaller home or a retirement community. At the end of the session, the CFT therapist told Lupé that she could call again in the future and come in for more therapy sessions if she encountered any difficulties with transitions in Julio's care needs. Lupé was grateful that the door remained open for her to come back if she needed to.

Pragmatic Issues in Practicing Caregiver Family Therapy

9

P rofessional service providers working with caregiving families of older adults encounter distinct challenges in managing the business, ethical, and financial as well as the clinical aspects of practice. This chapter uses a question-and-answer format to address commonly asked questions about how to implement caregiver family therapy (CFT) in practice settings.

Who Attends CFT Sessions?

Initial intakes are conducted with whoever initially seeks services (primary caregiver and/or other family members). Subsequent decisions about whom to include are determined jointly by the client and therapist. In cases in which the goal is to increase the support from secondary caregivers in the family, the therapist may wish to engage those members in

DOI: 10.1037/13943-009
Caregiver Family Therapy: Empowering Families to Meet the Challenges of Aging,
by S. H. Qualls and A. A. Williams

a joint session or, alternatively, to empower the primary caregiver to request support outside of a session as a deliberate strategy to build his or her skill and self-efficacy. In cases of unremitting family conflict over the nature of the problem, a joint session (electronic or live) is often very useful to allow the therapist to review the data carefully and respond to each person's concerns about the way the problem is being defined. Obviously, long-term family conflicts are unlikely to be resolved fully in the context of the immediate caregiving situation, as discussed in Chapter 4, so the decision about whom to include in ongoing CFT sessions requires thoughtful consideration of exactly whose involvement is relevant to the creation of a stable caregiving system. Other potential participants in CFT include other members of the caregiver's primary support network who may be key to supporting self-care activities.

The person seeking help is often, but not always, the primary caregiver. The identity of the help seeker influences therapeutic choices about whom should be included in the sessions and the focus of intervention. It also influences how the services are documented and billed.

A primary caregiver may seek services for himself or herself, or for others, such as the care recipient or the family as a whole. Caregivers who seek help for themselves may be focused initially on problem solving about care decisions or strategies or may ask for help dealing with caregiver distress or burden. Usually they attend the session alone. Regardless of initial presentation, a careful interview is likely to reveal that many of these requests reflect a level of distress that can be appropriately attributed to a mental disorder using existing coding systems (e.g., the *Diagnostic and Statistical Manual of Mental Disorders* [4th ed., text rev.], the *International Statistical Classification of Diseases and Related Health Problems* [10th rev.]) because the client actually reports symptoms. Occasionally, a caregiver will request primarily information or problem-solving help in the absence of symptoms, thus not qualifying for health insurance reimbursement. Long-term psychotherapy clients may become caregivers, requiring a shift in focus or at least positioning long-term clinical themes within the contexts of the caregiver role.

A client may ask you to see an older family member for a problem (e.g., depression), which should lead you to ask clarifying questions about the symptoms observed to ensure that you are an appropriate first help-seeking stop:

- Are there physical symptoms that worry you? (Difficulties with shortness of breath, heart palpitations, pain, or other potential indicators of physical illness should be evaluated by a primary care provider, or if urgent, an emergency care unit.)
- When was the older adult last examined by a health care provider?
- Is your loved one highly distressed or afraid of others trying to hurt him or her? Any indications of delusion or hallucination?

The initial name given to the problem is an interpretation or attribution for specific behaviors and may be inaccurate unless based on an appropriately thorough assessment. The initial telephone contact is a great time to ask the previous clarifying questions about whether you are the appropriate starting point for services (see Chapter 2). Some family members need to go straight to a physician for symptoms that could be biomedical in nature. If the symptoms have been evaluated recently, the therapist may request that the client bring certain medical reports to the first session to expedite the process of naming the problem. Other presenting problems suggest that the older adults' problem may be cognitive impairment. In such cases, the CFT therapist will want to tell the caregiver client that he or she should come to the first therapy session alone and that the older adult with cognitive impairment may be invited to future sessions to join the conversation.

In most cases in which multiple people in the family seek the service (e.g., daughter and mother who care for their father, sisters who care for a brother), they are working together to provide care at some level. One may be more reluctant to seek help than the others, and one may have an unspoken agenda for the others, but multiple members who agree to come to CFT usually have some common goal in mind. The siblings often want to form a plan to implement a decision they believe will not be popular with the older adult they love. They are simply trying to be on the same page, forming roles ahead of time that strengthen their ability to respond to strong resistance, for example.

Among clients who are not the primary caregiver, some are trying to figure out how to help the primary caregiver. A common example of the latter is an adult child who is worried about a parent caring for another parent. The same CFT processes are relevant because as a coach or guide, the therapist needs to understand the care recipient's problem as fully as possible before offering suggestions about the family's role structure to provide care. Ideally, a secondary caregiver could use CFT sessions to prepare for a joint session with the primary caregiver in which the options could be explored together. An advantage of a joint session is that the primary caregiver can inform the client of what is truly stressful and what is truly helpful to him or her, and the therapist can make an independent assessment of the level of distress or overwhelm that the primary caregiver is actually experiencing.

Other secondary caregiver clients are angry at the primary caregiver for a care-delivery choice, for example, when a sibling is upset at another sibling's caregiving behavior. The practical challenge is figuring out how to form an alliance with the person in the room while withholding judgment about how the family structure is, or is not, serving the care recipient well. The angry sibling client may be seeking validation from an authority to include in future arguments about why the client's preferred strategy is better or may genuinely want to work toward a better understanding with the primary caregiver so they can more effectively support each other and the care recipient.

Caregivers may also seek help to resolve conflict within the family. Highly conflicted families are unlikely to agree readily to come to therapy without some careful strategizing. The telephone contact may be too brief to allow the therapist to identify whether he or she prefers to have multiple family members come to the first session or not. Clients who request to bring other family members may be given an open welcome or may be asked a bit more about the rationale for bringing the others. Therapists usually find it very informative to watch a system in action. We usually allow the family to decide who shows up in the initial session and work from there.

Who Is the Client in CFT?

Often, at least one family member ends up as the primary person with whom the intervention is structured, with other family members joining for particular sessions, either live or via phone or e-connection. However, multiple family members may attend all sessions together, and the focus may be on their shared caregiving experience rather than on the care recipient per se. The decision about who is the client has implications for billing that are critical to consider. Here we simply note that if the help seeker is in distress and is going to receive services billed to health insurance, then that person must be the client. If the family is receiving service to assist an older adult with medical care, the client must be the care recipient according to Medicare rules. If multiple family members attend CFT together and pay privately, then the family may be the client.

All members attending a session must consent to services by signing a form that details the rules for services. Forms may be kept in a common file or in separate files, depending on how the service is conceptualized and how it is billed. Confidentiality rules to negotiate when multiple family members are involved are discussed later in this chapter.

How Do I Engage Distant Family Members Who Want to Be Involved?

Distant family members are often engaged in the work via conference call. Simple mechanisms of disseminating important information to relevant family members are commonly used. Fax, e-mail (secured only), or postal services can deliver medical or neuropsychological reports, care plans, and even values surveys that allow others to have input through writing.

Technologies allow for sharing communication or records. Video conferencing (e.g., via Skype) can be used to bring a person's face as well as voice into the room from a distance. Conference calls can include multiple persons. Some families maintain a personal health record for the care recipient online so that all approved family members can be afforded access to the records of health services (Blechman, 2009). Electronic communication systems are linking families with older adults using various platforms that are accessible even to persons who do not use computers (e.g., Williams & Lewis, 2009).

How Does the Structure of Each Session Flow?

CFT sessions in an outpatient environment are usually scheduled for 50 minutes if one to two people are attending, except for the intake session, which usually is scheduled for 90 minutes. Initial intake session(s) are focused on identifying the reason for help seeking at this time, along with information gathering, so are highly structured by the therapist to elicit key information. Subsequent sessions usually begin with reporting or updating on tasks the caregiver may have accomplished since the last session, followed by an agenda that focuses on moving through the steps of the model. In the final few minutes, the therapist typically summarizes the content of the session (and process, as relevant) and work with the client to identify next action steps.

CFT sessions offered in integrated care settings will be shaped by the culture and context. Primary care sessions are usually very brief, so CFT applications in that setting may happen in 15- to 20-minute sessions using brief interventions. The CFT therapist may rely on information gathered by other disciplines (e.g., nursing, social work) to understand the problems of the caregiver and/or care recipient. Relatively brief conversations may target very specific problems to be solved or specific points of resistance to implementing a care plan. In long-term-care settings, CFT frameworks or principles may be used during intermittent family visits for the purpose of helping them change their ways of interfacing with staff, residents, or each other. Care plan conferences can leverage attention to important changes that are needed. In legal and social service settings, CFT principles and strategies can be useful in family mediation activities. In short, CFT is a framework or model as well as a protocol, so it can be implemented flexibly in a variety of settings that constrain the length of sessions and the structure of sessions.

How Do I Schedule a Session Around Multiple Family Members' Schedules?

One of the trickier aspects of conducting family therapy with all-adult families is that the relevant members rarely live under the same roof or even in the same city. Flexibility is therefore key to scheduling larger family meetings. Holiday weekends, scheduled health events (e.g., surgery), and family reunions may be times the family is gathering naturally, and we often attempt to meet with them in conjunction with these natural visits. We sometimes schedule a longer session on a Saturday or evening to accommodate both our schedule and theirs.

Family sessions may be offered during holiday periods in an effort to make possible a meeting among multiple family members. One-shot sessions like that may require 1½ to 2 hours or more, depending on the goal of the meeting. Family sessions involving multiple people often require longer than 45 to 50 minutes unless a series of sessions are going to be used.

Whenever possible, empower the primary caregiver to ask for, and set up, the meeting that he or she needs with family members. The process of coaching the primary caregiver in accomplishing these tasks will be both informative about how the family system operates and an intervention designed to benefit the primary caregiver. E-mail often is an efficient way to work on scheduling for larger family meetings, but sometimes multiple contacts are needed before a meeting can be established.

Multiple family members in geographically dispersed families may need to connect more through e-mail or conference calls rather than in person. Careful consideration must be given to the reason that multiple people need to be included prior to designing the strategy for inclusion. For example, information sharing might be done asynchronously in time—caregiver sends today and gets response tomorrow. Slowing down communication sequences can help families avoid old automatic responses in favor of careful, deliberately chosen new communication patterns. Shared problem solving for a highly sensitive or urgent matter may require simultaneously timed communication (i.e., everyone is on the call together).

How Do I Deal With Stepfamily Conflicts?

Caregiving can be significantly more complex when stepfamilies are involved. Later life marriages may be strained when one member requires significant care from another frail spouse of only 5 or 10 years. In some families, the care recipients' adult children may disagree with the approach to care taken by the stepparent. In other families, even if the spouses are in good agreement about care services, adult children of the caregiver may resent the burden and stress placed on their parent by the needs of another parent.

Later life care often incurs significant cost that reduces the assets available for inheritance. Prenuptial agreements and wills can be used to specify the percentage of lifelong assets that will be assigned to a later life spouse versus the children from previous marriage(s). Regardless of such specifications, adult children sometimes become distressed when other family members or formal providers use the parent's assets for expensive end-of-life care because the overall size of the nest egg will be affected. In some cases, the children are blatantly greedy and appear to be uncaring for the parents. However, in other cases, a true difference of opinion about what constitutes good care can be influenced by fears about spending down the core asset pool. Even formal providers such as physicians or care managers may be the target of resentment from family members who lack any control over how their "future inheritance" is spent.

CFT therapists need a strong team of advisers for litigious situations, including an elder law attorney who knows the case law of recent years in which elder-care family battles have been litigated. The National Elder Law Attorney Association is a resource for finding a qualified attorney with whom to work. The probate section of the local Bar Association also likely offers continuing legal education classes or community forums that are a useful source of education for therapists new to these dilemmas.

Can I Bill Medicare for CFT?

Medicare pays for CFT services for two reasons: (a) to address mental health problems in the caregiver and (b) to assist family in meeting health needs of the care recipient. Thus, in order to bill Medicare, one needs to establish clearly in the record that the family intervention services are necessary for one of those two purposes.

Caregiver mental health needs must be established through an appropriate diagnostic procedure, and the billing must be done under that person's name. Education or coaching in effective caregiving methods would not likely meet Medicare's criteria for reimbursement as mental health services.

Care recipient health needs often require behavior changes on the part of other family members. The family often provides substantial health care in support of older adults, and sessions that address the family's needs to provide that support can be billed if the session includes both the caregiver(s) and care recipient. Family interventions without the patient present are not reimbursed by Medicare as of this writing.

If you plan to bill Medicare for services to families, you need to be particularly up-to-date on the rules from the Centers for Medicare and Medicaid Services (CMS) as well as the intermediary insurance agency that contracts with Medicare to handle claims. Both have rules that must be followed in order to avoid fraud. The American Psychological Association Practice Directorate also has information about Medicare compliance that can be a useful guide but does not supersede the rules generated by CMS and the intermediaries.

Whose Name Is on the Chart When Multiple People in the Family Are Seen?

The answer may depend on how you have structured the service. If the service is structured around a primary caregiver, you may have a single chart under the caregiver's name that includes session notes from larger family meetings that were designed to enhance support to him or her. If the service is structured around the care recipient, his or her name may be on the chart, and all subsequent services to families are documented as supportive of the care of the care recipient. If the service is set up at the beginning as family therapy and funded by sources other than health insurance (e.g., private pay or contract with a senior housing facility), you may have a family name on the file and include all sessions related to the family.

What Do I Do When a Family Member Demands Information About the Older Adult?

The intake process should clarify who in the family has access to what information about the care recipient and according to what legal authority. Starting with the consent-to-treat procedure, the therapist needs to clarify who his or her own legal decision maker is and who has a proxy decision maker. Some type of documentation is needed to afford any person access to health information about another person. Many families use a functional proxy decision maker without having clarified that authority legally so demand the right to information on the basis of their informally defined roles. Therapists need to clarify rights to information legally so cannot rely on informal family role structures.

What Issues Arise When Cognitive Impairment Limits a Family Member's Decision-Making Capacity?

Care recipients with cognitive impairment that renders their capacity for independent decisions questionable would have to be evaluated to determine the level of decision-making capacity, if that has not already been done. Therapists must become familiar with the state-sanctioned process for invoking a guardianship or durable power of attorney. Note that although care systems (e.g., hospitals, senior housing) have become more concerned about protecting privacy, therapists must meet the standards of their state and profession for documenting whether a person is considered to have, or not have, the capacity to make particular decisions. A record of evaluation and judgment by a qualified health care professional may be used, or if no formal documentation is available, the therapist needs to help the family initiate that process. Additional information about these issues and processes are addressed in the outstanding American Bar Association Commission on Law and Aging and American Psychological Association (2005) handbook *Assessment of Older Adults With Diminished Capacity* (available online at http:// www.apa.org/pi/aging/programs/assessment/capacity-psychologist-handbook.pdf).

Intake procedures need to clarify exactly who provides authority to the therapist to talk with whom about what information over what period of time. A consent-to-disclose document needs to be completed and signed at that time to provide legal authority for the therapist to ask or tell any information about a client to anyone.

Many resources are now available to therapists working with older adults whose decisional capacity is in question. Therapists need to learn the lay of the land in the legal world (Marshall, Seal, & Vanatta-Perry, 2007; Moye & Braun, 2007; Qualls, 2007b) as well as the background literature on factors that constrain capacity (Kaye & Grigsby, 2007; Wood & Tanius, 2007). Guidelines and frameworks for clinical procedures that assess capacity related to particular functional domains such as finances and medical consent are available (Hebert & Marson, 2007; Moye & Braun, 2007; Wood & Tanius, 2007), as are intervention approaches to enhance capacity to participate to the fullest possible level (Qualls, 2007a). As noted previously, the American Bar Association Commission on Law and Aging and the American Psychological Association (2005, 2006, 2008) have collaborated on outstanding guidebooks for lawyers, judges, and psychologists.

How Can I Handle the Situation When Family Members Want to Talk on the Phone Between Sessions About Other Participants in Therapy?

Practical questions such as the following need to be asked when one family member wants to speak privately with the therapist about other family members:

- Why do you want to tell me this now rather than in the room with other family members?
- What do you want me to do with this information?
- How does this revelation relate to the initial rules of confidentiality and information sharing that were negotiated early in therapy?

Family secrets are a perennial challenge in family therapy (Imber-Black, 1993). Although there may be legitimate reasons for sharing a piece of information privately, the privacy also can function to position the sharer with power. An example of a legitimate reason is when a caregiver does not want to humiliate or distress a care recipient by detailing his or her difficulties in front of others. In some cases, the therapist will simply ask the caller to schedule a private session to discuss concerns. In other cases, however, the therapist may choose to avoid risking breach of trust with one member by having a private session with another. Regardless of the therapeutic decision, expectations must be clarified about exactly what will happen to this information shared outside the context of other therapy participants' hearing.

How Do I Work With Other Disciplines?

Often and gratefully. Rarely can therapists provide all of the assessment and intervention needed in complex elder-care cases. With the client(s)' legally assigned authority, the therapist likely will obtain and share information regularly with other disciplines, including primary care providers, specialty health providers, care managers, home health staff, residential facility staff, and so on.

Typically, therapists are functioning on a virtual team with other providers, without the benefit of knowing who is on the team or what their care plan might be. One way to improve that care coordination nightmare is to obtain consent in initial meetings to contact the key care providers involved with the care recipient and caregiver. A template form that lists providers by discipline can be used to elicit information about who is on the virtual team. For example, a listing of disciplines might offer the option of checking off those involved in care, with a blank to fill in with the person's name and contact information. The right to contact each person must be clearly authorized for a particular purpose in a particular time frame. Once authorized to be in contact, therapists can use faxed requests for information, secure e-mail services, or telephone contacts to elicit and share appropriate information.

Therapists would do well to honor the very busy schedules of all professionals and ask for or share information only when it is targeted to a particular use. We find it helpful to tell someone why we are giving them, or requesting from them, information. We also use ancillary staff or faxed requests as much as possible so we can minimize demands on very busy professionals for clerical work. Furthermore, a faxed request for a phone call, e-mail access (only some health providers offer this option), or any action is more likely to be visible than a note about a telephone call. We encourage keeping a clear paper trail of your requests and making each request very clear. In short, CFT therapists need to prepare families to work effectively within the work flow of various care systems.

What Do I Do When Family Members Might Be Abusing an Older Person?

State laws are quite specific about the duty of practitioners to report abuse. Almost all states require helping professionals of all types to report any suspected abuse. States vary on which helping professionals are named, the standards for evidence needed to invoke required reporting, and the required reporting process. Professionals are simply required to know state statutes and follow them.

As with all family interventions, reporting abuse is likely to alter the relationship between client and therapist. Clients may feel betrayed when a therapist reports, but they may also feel grateful. Therapists must stay clear at all times with clients about what must be reported, not only in the intake sessions when the legal consent-to-inform documents are signed but also at the time that information is shared. Therapists can sometimes convince the family to make the report if it appears they might gain more control in some way by being the reporter. We find that we can often salvage the therapeutic relationship by communicating clearly with the client about what is going to happen, how it can be used to improve the care recipient's life, and how the therapist will proceed to work with the family during the period of investigation. Regardless, therapists have no choice and must proceed to report abuse even if the relationship is lost.

Therapists who work within formal care settings (e.g., housing) in which a staff member is suspected of abuse also need to attend to the rules of the facility or agency. No agency or facility rule can absolve therapists of their reporting responsibilities. But in addition to formal reporting, a therapist may want to work with the management team and staff to use the incident to educate, build the team's competence and comfort with mutual support, and form a plan for dealing with the fallout from family members and other residents. Likely, a complex series of reactions will unfold within the setting, which the therapist may be asked to help manage. The family is unlikely to be asked to pay for those services; the agency or facility should be the pay source for services designed to help it.

We find it valuable to maintain a positive, collaborative relationship with the Adult Protective Services (APS) staff within the county human services agency because they are the ultimate family safety net. When poor care is being provided, and our best efforts with the family have not yielded effective action, APS may be our best leverage point. Families rightfully fear losing basic decision-making rights over their members, so they may become engaged in more protective action if they understand that the poor care requires the therapist (or others) to report potential abuse or neglect.

When the Care Recipient Lives in Another State or Region, How Can I Help my Client?

Every U.S. region has an Area Agency on Aging (AAA) that offers information and assistance and contracts for a wide range of other services.

Finding the local AAA is remarkably easy online at http://www.elder-care.gov. You insert the zip code of the care recipient's home and will be provided contact information for the nearest AAA. Some AAAs offer direct caregiver support services, and others contract out services to other agencies. Regardless, the AAA can be expected to provide listings of local resources (health care, housing, social services), and can direct families to family support resources.

A wide range of other community resource agencies and organizations offer information and support to families. Some states also offer state-funded resource organizations (e.g., California has Alzheimer's Resource Centers that are very useful to families dealing with cognitive impairment). Illness-specific advocacy organizations also have regional or local offices that offer resource and referrals for services to families caring for persons with those conditions (e.g., Alzheimer's Association, Stroke Association, American Heart Association). Libraries often have resource centers for disease-specific as well as general caregiving informational needs. Land-grant universities have extension offices that often provide outreach on aging-specific care concerns. The concept of "no wrong door" that is driving current policy is helping agencies work together to direct families where they need to go, regardless of which door they enter first to see help.

Where Can I Get Additional Resources for Serving Caregivers?

Websites such as the following offer rich repositories of guidance and resources for therapists wishing to work with caregivers:

- The American Psychological Association's Caregiver Briefcase website: http://www.apa.org/pi/about/publications/caregivers/index.aspx
- Family Caregiver Alliance: http://www.caregiver.org
- Family Caregiving 101 (National Family Caregivers Association and the National Alliance for Caregiving), http://www.familycaregiving101.org
- Family Care Resource Clearinghouse (AXA Foundation and National Alliance for Caregiving): http://web.raffa.com/nac/axa/
- National Alliance for Caregiving: http://www.caregiving.org
- National Caregivers Library (FamilyCare America): http://www.caregiverslibrary.org
- National Family Caregiving Association: http://www.nfcacares.org
- Strength for Caring (Johnson & Johnson): http://www.strengthforcaring.com

■ The Department of Veterans Affairs' six-module training guide for family caregivers of veterans of any age: http://www.caregiver.va.gov/support_workbook.asp

What Does the Affordable Care Act (ACA) of 2010 Offer Caregivers?

Long-term services and supports for persons with disabilities and chronic conditions, which are highly relevant to caregivers of older adults, are addressed in the Affordable Care Act (ACA) of 2010 with funds to states to improve services access and choice. Support is targeted toward the five key characteristics of a high-performing support system for families of older adults: support for family caregivers, ease of access and affordability, choice of settings and providers, quality of care and life, and effective transitions and organization of care (Reinhard, Kassner, & Houser, 2011). The ACA adds financial incentives to states to balance funding of institutional care with home-based care through programs such as Money Follows the Person and Community First Choice. Additional funding for Aging and Disability Resource Centers enhances their capacity to link with the variety of places in which families seek service in support of the no wrong door concept that allows families to end up in the right place regardless of where they start. Policy shifts toward family-friendly and family-supportive long-term services and supports are likely to continue to support family choice in caregiving contexts and services because they are quite simply cost-effective.

How Do I Manage the Emotional Demands of Family Therapy Work, Especially When it Mirrors my Personal Family Life Experiences?

Family therapy has a tradition of observation-based consultation or supervision that is particularly helpful to keep the therapist aware of the potential fuzzy boundaries between personal and professional. CFT therapists can benefit from continuing that tradition in which work is observed occasionally as well. Even trainees who are perhaps most anxious about being observed making mistakes eventually learn that observation is their best friend because observers almost always bring new ideas to the work.

The processes outlined in these chapters ultimately describe an approach to family therapy that is applied to unique family contexts, situated near the end of life for many of the family members involved. Particular challenges for CFT therapists include working with systems (e.g., families, health care, social services, virtual teams), working with individuals and families contending with chronic health conditions and cognitive impairment, and thereby dealing with loss of functioning and death. These families face their own histories, present realities, and futures.

Like other family therapies, CFT evokes in the therapist strong feelings about family dynamics and difficult aging dilemmas. Practicing CFT may, on occasion, require the therapist to spend time in personal psychotherapy or family therapy examining issues in his or her own family of origin (Framo, 1992). Our own personal history within our own family is so potent that therapeutic work with families almost inevitably pushes our buttons at one point or another. Given that most therapists will go through their own parent-care challenges during midlife, the probability is high that therapist and client will share some of the same parent-care or spouse-care issues, concerns, and even family dynamics. CFT therapists must take particular care and pay particular attention to keep on top of their reactions to clients' family dilemmas. Indeed, therapists must put effort into their own self-care in order to maintain the resilience they are promoting in their caregiver clients.

CFT also brings us face to face with human mortality and how difficult the journey can be along the way. Clients sometimes spell out graphic details about diseases and dying processes as part of their effort to make meaning. Therapists can be traumatized if they have not worked through their own fears of death and dying. As with mental health work with older adults, young adult trainees are facing these existentially potent challenges off time in their own development, often decades before their parents will be burdened with chronic disease (Knight, 2004). On the other hand, trainees and experienced therapists bring their own life pains into the room and thus are vulnerable to reexperiencing difficult times within their own relationship networks when disease or death claimed or complicated the lives of people they love.

In short, family therapy is always evocative, and family therapy with chronic illness at the end of life is doubly so. We hope those reading this book have gained frameworks, skills, and strategies for handling some of life's most challenging dilemmas and existentially meaningful experiences. We hope our clients' stories offer hope, guidance, and encouragement to share the richness of life's journey at a point in the life span that is still largely uncharted territory within families.

Appendix A
Caregiver Reaction Scale

T he following questions are designed to help us understand the types of difficulties you and your family face as caregivers.

Each item is ranked on a 1 to 4 scale.

1 (not at all)   2 (somewhat)   3 (quite a bit)   4 (completely)

<u>Please respond to all items by checking (√) the appropriate box</u>

(A) *Here are some thoughts and feelings that people sometimes have about themselves as caregivers. How much does each statement describe your thoughts about your caregiving:*

	1	2	3	4
Wish you were free to lead a life of your own				
Feel trapped by your relative's illness				
Wish you could just run away				
Feel stressed by your relative's illness and needs				

(B) *How much does each statement describe you:*

	1	2	3	4
You are exhausted when you go to bed at night				
You have more to do than you can handle				
You don't have time just for yourself				
You work hard as a caregiver but never seem to make any progress				

(C) *Caregivers sometimes feel that they lose important things in life because of their relative's illness. To what extent have you personally lost the following:*

	1	2	3	4
Being able to confide in your relative				
The person whom you used to know				
Having someone who really knew you well				
A chance to do some of the things you planned				
Contact with other people				
A sense of who you are				
Lost an important part of yourself				

(D) *People can often learn things about themselves from taking care of a relative. How much do you:*

	1	2	3	4
Believe you've learned how to deal with this very difficult situation				
Feel that, all in all, you're a good caregiver				
In general, feel competent as a caregiver				
Feel self-confident as a caregiver				

(E) *Since becoming a caregiver, how much have you:*

	1	2	3	4
Become more aware of your inner strengths				
Become more self-confident				
Grown as a person				
Learned to do things you didn't do before				

(F) *There are many different ways of coping with the stress of caregiving. How often do you:*

	1	2	3	4
Try to accept your relative as he/she is, not how you wish he/she could be				
Try to think about the present rather than the future				

Try to keep your sense of humor				
Spend time alone				
Eat				
Smoke				
Get some exercise				
Watch TV				
Read				
Take some medication to calm you down				
Drink some alcohol				

(G) *Family members don't always see eye-to-eye when it comes to dealing with a relative who is ill. How much disagreement have you had with anyone in your family about the following issues:*

	1	2	3	4
The seriousness of your relative's memory problems				
The need to watch out for your relative's safety				
What things your relative is able to do for himself/herself				
Whether your relative should be placed in a nursing home or assisted living				

(H) *How much disagreement have you had with people in your family because they:*

	1	2	3	4
Don't spend enough time with your relative				
Don't do their share in caring for your relative				
Don't show enough respect for your relative				
Lack patience with your relative				
Don't visit or telephone you enough				
Don't give you enough help				
Don't show enough appreciation for your work as a caregiver				
Give you unwanted advice				

(I) *How much do you agree with the following statements about your present work situation:*

	1	2	3	4
You have less energy for your work				
You have missed too many days				
You have been dissatisfied with the quality of your work				
You worry about your relative while you're at work				
Phone calls about or from your relative interrupt your work				

(J) *These questions ask about your household expenses and your standard of living. Compared with just before you began to take care of your relative, how much would you agree with the following statements:*

	1	2	3	4
Total household income has decreased				
Total monthly expenses have increased				
In general, family finances work out at the end of the month				

_____   _____

Name of person completing form   **Date**

Appendix B
Summary of the Caregiver Family Therapy Process

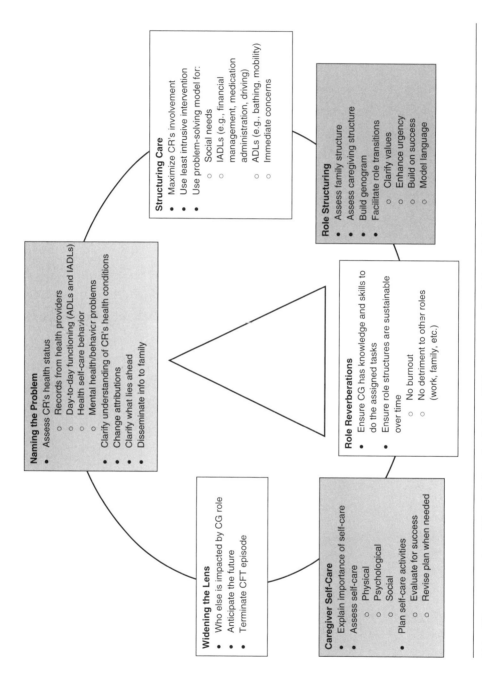

Naming the Problem
- Assess CR's health status
  - Records from health providers
  - Day-to-day functioning (ADLs and IADLs)
  - Health self-care behavior
  - Mental health/behavior problems
- Clarify understanding of CR's health conditions
- Change attributions
- Clarify what lies ahead
- Disseminate info to family

Structuring Care
- Maximize CR's involvement
- Use least intrusive intervention
- Use problem-solving model for:
  - Social needs
  - IADLs (e.g., financial management, medication administration, driving)
  - ADLs (e.g., bathing, mobility)
  - Immediate concerns

Role Structuring
- Assess family structure
- Assess caregiving structure
- Build genogram
- Facilitate role transitions
  - Clarify values
  - Enhance urgency
  - Build on success
  - Model language

Role Reverberations
- Ensure CG has knowledge and skills to do the assigned tasks
- Ensure role structures are sustainable over time
  - No burnout
  - No detriment to other roles (work, family, etc.)

Widening the Lens
- Who else is impacted by CG role
- Anticipate the future
- Terminate CFT episode

Caregiver Self-Care
- Explain importance of self-care
- Assess self-care
  - Physical
  - Psychological
  - Social
- Plan self-care activities
  - Evaluate for success
  - Revise plan when needed

Note. CR = care recepient; ADL = Activities of daily living; IADL = instrumental activities of daily living; CG = caregiver.

References

Acierno, R., Hernandez, M., Amstadter, A., Resnick, H., Steve, K., Muzzy, W., & Kilpatrick, D. (2010). Prevalence and correlates of emotional, physical, sexual, and financial abuse and potential neglect in the United States: The national elder mistreatment study. *American Journal of Public Health, 100*, 292–297. doi:10.2105/AJPH.2009.163089

Acton, G. J. (2002). Health-promoting self-care in family caregivers. *Western Journal of Nursing Research, 24*, 73–86. doi:10.1177/01939450222045716

American Bar Association Commission on Law and Aging and American Psychological Association. (2005). *Assessment of older adults with diminished capacity: A handbook for lawyers*. Washington, DC: Author.

American Bar Association Commission on Law and Aging and American Psychological Association. (2006). *Judicial determination of capacity of older adults in guardianship proceedings: A handbook for judges*. Washington, DC: Author.

American Bar Association Commission on Law and Aging and American Psychological Association. (2008). *Assessment of older adults with diminished capacity: A handbook for psychologists*. Washington, DC: Author.

American Psychological Association. (Producer). (2006). *Treating alzheimer's disease through caregiver family therapy* [DVD]. Available from http://www.apa.org/pubs/videos

American Psychological Association. (2012). Guidelines for the evaluation of dementia and age-related cognitive change. *American Psychologist, 67*, 1–9. doi:10.1037/a0024643

Anderson, L. N. (2011). *Attributions and symptom reports of cognitive impairment: Testing the symmetry rule in caregiver therapy clients.* Unpublished doctoral dissertation, University of Colorado, Colorado Springs.

Anderson, L. N., Horning, S., June, A., Kane, K., Marty, M., Pepin, R., & Vair, C. (2008). *The Aging Families and Caregiver Program: A guide to caregiver family therapy.* Unpublished manuscript.

Aneshensel, C. S., Pearlin, L. I., Mullan, J. T., Zarit, S. H., & Whitlatch, C. J. (1995). *Profiles in caregiving: The unexpected career.* San Diego, CA: Academic Press.

Annon, J. F. (1974). *The behavioral treatment of sexual problems.* Honolulu, HI: Enabling Systems.

Antonucci, T. C. (1986). Hierarchical mapping technique. *Generations: Journal of the American Society on Aging, 10*(4), 10–12.

Aquilino, W. S. (2006). Family relationships and support systems in early adulthood. In J. J. Arnett & J. L. Tanner (Eds.), *Emerging adults in America: Coming of age in the 21st century* (pp. 193–217). Washington, DC: American Psychological Association. doi:10.1037/11381-008

Areán, P., Hegel, M., Vannoy, S., Fan, M., & Unuzter, J. (2008). Effectiveness of problem-solving therapy for older, primary care patients with depression: Results from the IMPACT Project. *The Gerontologist, 48*, 311–323. doi:10.1093/geront/48.3.311

Arnett, J. J. (2004). *Emerging adulthood: The winding road from the late teens through the twenties.* New York, NY: Oxford University Press.

Ayalon, L., Bornfeld, H., Gum, A. M., & Areán, P. A. (2008). The use of problem-solving therapy and restraint-free environment for the management of depression and agitation in long-term care. *Clinical Gerontologist, 32*, 77–90. doi:10.1080/07317110802468728

Baltes, P. B., & Baltes, M. M. (1990). Psychological perspectives on successful aging: The model of selective optimization with compensation. In P. B. Baltes & M. M. Baltes (Eds.), *Successful aging: Perspectives from the behavioral sciences* (pp. 1–34). Cambridge, England: Cambridge University Press. doi:10.1017/CBO9780511665684.003

Baltes, P. B., Lindenberger, U., & Staudinger, U. M. (2006). Life span theory in developmental psychology. In R. M. Lerner & W. Damon (Eds.), *Handbook of child psychology: Vol. 1. Theoretical models of human development* (6th ed., pp. 569–664). Hoboken, NJ: Wiley.

Bandura, A. (1977). Self-efficacy: Toward a unifying theory of behavioral change. *Psychological Review, 84*, 191–215. doi:10.1037/0033-295X.84.2.191

Beck, A. T., & Alford, B. A. (2009). *Depression: Causes and treatment* (2nd ed.). Baltimore, MD: University of Pennsylvania Press.

Beck, C. M., & Ferguson, D. (1981). Aged abuse. *Journal of Gerontological Nursing, 7*, 333–336.

Belle, S. H., Burgio, L., Burns, R., Coon, D., Czaja, S. J., Gallagher-Thompson, D., . . . Zhang, S. (2006). Enhancing the quality of life of dementia caregivers from different ethnic or racial groups: A randomized controlled trial. *Annals of Internal Medicine, 145,* 727–738.

Blechman, E. A. (2009). Personal health records for older adults with chronic conditions and their informal caregivers. In S. H. Qualls & S. H. Zarit (Eds.), *Aging families and caregiving* (pp. 287–310). Hoboken, NJ: Wiley.

Blenkner, M. (1965). Social work and family relationships in later life with some thoughts on filial maturity. In E. Shanas & G. Streib (Eds.), *Social structure and the family: Generational relations* (pp. 46–59). Englewood Cliffs, NJ: Prentice-Hall.

Blieszner, R. (2009). Who are the aging families? In S. H. Qualls & S. H. Zarit (Eds.), *Aging families and caregiving* (pp. 1–18). Hoboken, NJ: Wiley.

Boise, L., Morgan, D., Kaye, J., & Camicioli, R. (1999). Delays in the diagnosis of dementia: Perspectives of family caregivers. *American Journal of Alzheimer's Disease and Other Dementias, 14,* 20–26. doi:10.1177/153331759901400101

Boss, P., Caron, W., Horbal, J., & Mortimer, J. (1990). Predictors of depression in caregivers of dementia patients: Boundary ambiguity and mastery. *Family Process, 29,* 245–254. doi:10.1111/j.1545-5300.1990.00245.x

Boss, P., & Greenberg, J. S. (1984). Family boundary ambiguity: A new variable in family stress theory. *Family Process, 23,* 535–546. doi:10.1111/j.1545-5300.1984.00535.x

Boszormenyi-Nagy, I., & Spark, G. M. (1984). *Invisible loyalties: Reciprocity in intergenerational family therapy.* New York, NY: Brunner/Mazel.

Bowen, M. (1978). *Family therapy in clinical practice.* New York, NY: Aronson.

Burns, D. D. (1999). *The feeling good handbook* (Rev. ed.). New York, NY: Plume/Penguin Books.

Cacioppo, J. T., Poehlmann, K. M., Kiecolt-Glaser, J. K., Malarkey, W. B., Burleson, M. H., Berntson, G. G., & Glaser, R. (1998). Cellular immune responses to acute stress in female caregivers of dementia patients and matched controls. *Health Psychology, 17,* 182–189. doi:10.1037/0278-6133.17.2.182

Carter, E. A., & McGoldrick, M. (Eds.). (1989). *The changing family life cycle: A framework for family therapy* (2nd ed.). New York, NY: Allyn & Bacon.

Chatters, L. M., Jayakody, R., & Taylor, R. J. (1994). Fictive kinship relations in black extended families. *Journal of Comparative Family Studies, 25,* 297–312.

Choi, N. G., & Mayer, J. (2000). Elder abuse, neglect, and exploitation: Risk factors and prevention strategies. *Journal of Gerontological Social Work, 33,* 5–25. doi:10.1300/J083v33n02_02

Coon, D. W., Gallagher-Thompson, D., & Thompson, L. W. (2003). *Innovative interventions to reduce dementia caregiver distress.* New York, NY: Springer.

Cooper, C., Blanchard, M., Sclwood, A., Walker, Z., & Livingston, J. (2010). Family carers' distress and abusive behavior. *The British Journal of Psychiatry, 196,* 480–485. doi:10.1192/bjp.bp.109.071811

Crowther, M., & Austin, A. (2009). The cultural context of clinical work with aging caregivers. In S. H. Qualls & S. H. Zarit (Eds.), *Aging families and caregiving* (pp. 45–60). Hoboken, NJ: Wiley.

Derogatis, L. R., & Melisaratos, N. (1983). The Brief Symptom Inventory: An introductory report. *Psychological Medicine, 13,* 595–605. doi:10.1017/S0033291700048017

Dessin, C. L. (2000). Financial abuse of the elderly. *Idaho Law Review, 36,* 203–226.

Dilworth-Anderson, P., & Gibson, B. (2002). The cultural influence of values, norms, meanings, and perceptions in understanding dementia in ethnic minorities. *Alzheimer Disease and Associated Disorders, 16,* S56–S63. doi:10.1097/00002093-200200002-00005

Doherty, W., & Baird, M. (1983). *Family therapy and family medicine.* New York, NY: Guilford Press.

Ducharme, F., & Levesque, L. Gendron, M., Leguat, A., Ward, J., & Trudeau, D. (2003). *Taking care of myself: An intervention program for caregivers of an institutionalized cognitively impaired elderly family member* (Facilitator's workbook). Montreal, Canada: Institut universitaire de geiatrie de Montreal, Centre de rechereché.

D'Zurilla, T. J., & Goldfried, M. R. (1971). Problem solving and behavior modification. *Journal of Abnormal Psychology, 78,* 107–126. doi:10.1037/h0031360

D'Zurilla, T. J., Nezu, A. M., & Maydeu-Olivares, A. (2004). Social problem-solving: Theory and assessment. In E. C. Chang, T. J. D'Zurilla, & L. J. Sanna (Eds.), *Social problem solving: Theory, research, and training* (pp. 11–27). Washington, DC: American Psychological Association. doi:10.1037/10805-001

Eisdorfer, C., Czaja, S. J., Loewenstein, D. A., Robert, M. P., Argüelles, S., Mitraani, V. B., & Szapocznik, J. (2003). The effect of a family therapy and technology-based intervention on caregiver depression. *The Gerontologist, 43,* 521–531. doi:10.1093/geront/43.4.521

Engel, G. L. (1980). The clinical application of the biopsychosocial model. *The American Journal of Psychiatry, 137,* 535–544.

Feil, N. (1993). *The validation breakthrough: Simple techniques for communicating with people with "Alzheimer's-type dementia."* Baltimore, MD: Health Professions Press.

Figley, C. (Ed.). (1998). *Burnout in families: The systemic costs of caring.* Boca Raton, FL: CRC Press.

Fingerman, K., Miller, L., & Seidel, A. (2009). Functions families serve in old age. In S. H. Qualls & S. H. Zarit (Eds.), *Aging families and caregiving* (pp. 19–43). Hoboken, NJ: Wiley.

Fiori, K. L., Antonucci, T. C., & Cortina, K. S. (2006). Social network typologies and mental health among older adults. *The Journals of Gerontology, Series B: Psychological Sciences, 61,* P25–P32. doi:10.1093/geronb/61.1.P25

Fisher, L., & Lieberman, M. A. (1996). The effects of family context on adult offspring of patients with Alzheimer's disease: A longitudinal study. *Journal of Family Psychology, 10,* 180–191. doi:10.1037/0893-3200.10.2.180

Folstein, M. F., Folstein, S. E., & McHugh, P. R. (1975). Mini-mental state: A practical method for grading the cognitive state of patients for the clinician. *Journal of Psychiatric Research, 12,* 189–198.

Framo, J. L. (1992). *Family-of-origin therapy: An intergenerational approach.* New York, NY: Brunner/Mazel.

Frankel, R. M., Quill, T. E., & McDaniel, S. H. (2003). *The biopsychosocial approach: Past, present, and future.* Rochester, NY: University of Rochester Press.

Fung, H. H., & Carstensen, L. L. (2004). Motivational changes in response to blocked goals and foreshortened time: Testing alternatives to socioemotional selectivity theory. *Psychology and Aging, 19,* 68–78. doi:10.1037/0882-7974.19.1.68

Gabriel, M. S. (2011). Trajectories of chronic illness. In S. H. Qualls & J. E. Kasl-Godley (Eds.), *End-of-life issues, grief, and bereavement* (pp. 26–42). Hoboken, NJ: Wiley.

Gallagher-Thompson, D., & Coon, D. W. (2007). Evidence-based psychological treatments for distress in family caregivers of older adults. *Psychology and Aging, 22,* 37–51. doi:10.1037/0882-7974.22.1.37

Gaugler, J. E., Hanna, N., Linder, J., Given, C. W., Tolbert, V., Kataria, R., & Regine, W. F. (2005). Cancer caregiving and subjective stress: A multi-site, multidimensional analysis. *Psycho-Oncology, 14,* 771–785. doi:10.1002/pon.916

Gaugler, J. E., Jarrott, S. E., Zarit, S. H., Parris Stephens, M., Townsend, A., & Greene, R. (2003). Respite for dementia caregivers: The effects of adult day service use on caregiving hours and care demands. *International Psychogeriatrics, 15,* 37–58. doi:10.1017/S1041610203008743

Gaugler, J. E., & Zarit, S. H. (2001). The effectiveness of adult day services for disabled older people. *Journal of Aging & Social Policy, 12,* 23–47. doi:10.1300/J031v12n02_03

Gerson, R. (1995). The family life cycle: Phases, stages, and crises. In R. H. Mikesell, D. D. Lusterman, & S. H. McDaniel (Eds.), *Integrating family therapy: Handbook of family psychology and systems theory* (pp. 91–111). Washington, DC: American Psychological Association. doi:10.1037/10172-005

Gilbert, D. T., & Malone, P. S. (1995). The correspondence bias. *Psychological Bulletin, 117,* 21–38. doi:10.1037/0033-2909.117.1.21

Gitlin, L. N., Winter, L., Corcoran, M., Dennis, M., Schinfeld, S., & Hauck, W. (2003). Effects of the Home Environmental Skill-Building Program on the caregiver-care recipient dyad: Six-month outcomes from the Philadelphia REACH Initiative. *The Gerontologist, 43,* 532–546. doi:10.1093/geront/43.4.532

Gitlin, L. N., Winter, L., & Dennis, M. P. (2010). Assistive devices caregivers use and find helpful to manage problem behaviors of dementia. *Gerontechnology, 9,* 408–414. doi:10.4017/gt.2010.09.03.006.00

Global Health Observatory. (2009). *Health care costs, a primer: Key information on health care costs and their impact.* Menlo Park, CA: The Henry J. Kaiser Family Foundation. Retrieved from http://www.kff.org/insurance/upload/7670_02.pdf

Glymour, M. M., & Manly, J. J. (2008). Lifecourse social conditions and racial and ethnic patterns of cognitive aging. *Neuropsychology Review, 18,* 223–254. doi:10.1007/s11065-008-9064-z

Gompertz, P., Pound, P., & Ebrahim, S. (1994). Validity of the extended activities of daily living scale. *Clinical Rehabilitation, 8,* 275–280. doi:10.1177/026921559400800401

Grossman, A. H., D'Augelli, A. R., & Dragowski, E. A. (2007). Caregiving and care receiving among older lesbian, gay, and bisexual adults. *Journal of Gay & Lesbian Social Services, 18,* 15–38. doi:10.1300/J041v18n03_02

Hafemeister, T. L. (2003). Financial abuse of the elderly in domestic situations. In R. J. Bonnie & R. B. Wallace (Eds.), *Elder mistreatment: Abuse, neglect, and exploitation in an aging America* (pp. 382–445). Washington, DC: National Academies Press.

Hagestad, G. O. (1986). The aging society as a context for family life. *Daedalus, 115,* 119–139.

Hagestad, G. O. (1988). Demographic change and the life course: Some emerging trends in the family realm. *Family Relations, 37,* 405–410. doi:10.2307/584111

Hargrave, T. D., & Anderson, W. T. (1992). *Finishing well: Aging and reparation in the intergenerational family.* New York, NY: Brunner/Mazel.

Hebert, K. R., & Marson, D. C. (2007). Assessment of financial capacity in older adults with dementia. In S. H. Qualls & M. A. Smyer (Eds.), *Changes in decision-making capacity in older adults: Assessment and intervention* (pp. 237–270). Hoboken, NJ: Wiley.

Henry, S., & Convery, A. (2006). *The eldercare handbook: Difficult choices, compassionate solutions.* New York, NY: Harper Collins.

Hikoyeda, N., Mukoyama, W. K., Liou, J. D., & Masterson, B. (2006). Working with Japanese American families. In G. Yeo & D. Gallagher-Thompson (Eds.), *Ethnicity and the dementias* (2nd ed., pp. 231–244). New York, NY: Routledge.

Houts, P. S., Nezu, A. M., Nezu, C. M., & Bucher, J. A. (1996). The prepared family caregiver: A problem-solving approach to family caregiver education. *Patient Education and Counseling, 27,* 63–73. doi:10.1016/0738-3991(95)00790-3

Howland, R. H. (2010). Drug theories for cognitive impairment and dementia. *Journal of Psychological Nursing, 48*(4), 11–14.

Imber-Black, E. (1993). *Secrets in families and family therapy.* New York, NY: Norton.

Jones, P. (1996). Adult protection work: The stories behind the statistics. *Aging Magazine, 367,* 19–24.

Jones, S. H. (2007). Self-care in caregiving. *Journal of Human Behavior in the Social Environment, 14,* 95–115. doi:10.1300/J137v14n01_05

Kaye, K., & Grigsby, J. (2007). Medical factors affecting mental capacity. In S. H. Qualls & M. A. Smyer (Eds.), *Changes in decision-making capacity in older adults: Assessment and intervention* (pp. 61–89). Hoboken, NJ: Wiley.

Kiecolt-Glaser, J. K., Dura, J. R., Speicher, C. E., Trask, O. J., & Glaser, R. (1991). Spousal caregivers of dementia victims: Longitudinal changes in immunity and health. *Psychosomatic Medicine, 53,* 345–362.

Kiecolt-Glaser, J. K., Glaser, R., Shuttleworth, E. C., Dyer, C. S., Ogrocki, P., & Speicher, C. E. (1987). Chronic stress and immunity in family caregivers of Alzheimer's disease victims. *Psychosomatic Medicine, 49,* 523–535.

Knight, B. G. (2004). *Psychotherapy with older adults.* Thousand Daks, CA: Sage.

Knight, B. G., & Losada, A. (2011). Family caregiving for cognitively or physically frail older adults: Theory, research, and practice. In K. W. Schaie & S. L. Willis (Eds.), *Handbook of the psychology of aging* (7th ed., pp. 353–365). San Diego, CA: Elsevier Academic Press. doi:10.1016/B978-0-12-380882-0.00023-1

Knight, B. G., & Sayegh, P. (2010). Cultural values and caregiving: The updated sociocultural stress and coping model. *The Journals of Gerontology, Series B: Psychological Sciences and Social Sciences, 65B,* 5–13. doi:10.1093/geronb/gbp096

Knopman, D., Donohue, J. A., & Gutterman, E. M. (2000). Patterns of care in the early stages of Alzheimer's disease: Impediments to timely diagnosis. *Journal of the American Geriatrics Society, 48,* 300–304.

Lai, D. W. L. (2010). Filial piety, caregiving appraisal, and caregiving burden. *Research on Aging, 32,* 200–223. doi:10.1177/0164027509351475

Lawton, M. P., & Brody, E. M. (1969). Assessment of older people: Self-maintaining and instrumental activities of daily living. *The Gerontologist, 9,* 179–186. doi:10.1093/geront/9.3_Part_1.179

LeBlanc, L. A., Cherup, S. M., Feliciano, L., & Sidener, T. M. (2006). Using choice-making opportunities to increase activity engagement in individuals with dementia. *American Journal of Alzheimer's Disease and Other Dementias, 21,* 318–325. doi:10.1177/1533317506292183

Leech, N. L., & Onwuegbuzie, A. J. (2007). An array of qualitative data analysis tools: A call for data analysis triangulation. *School Psychology Quarterly, 22,* 557–584. doi:10.1037/1045-3830.22.4.557

Leventhal, H., Brissette, I., & Leventhal, E. (2003). The common-sense model of self-regulation of health and illness. In L. D. Cameron & H. Leventhal (Eds.), *The self-regulation of health and illness behavior* (pp. 42–65). New York, NY: Routledge.

Lieberman, M. A., & Fisher, L. (1999). The effects of family conflict resolution and decision making on the provision of help for an elder with Alzheimer's disease. *The Gerontologist, 39,* 159–166. doi:10.1093/geront/39.2.159

Liu, W., & Gallagher-Thompson, D. (2009). Impact of dementia caregiving: Risks, strains, and growth. In S. H. Qualls & S. H. Zarit (Eds.), *Aging families and caregiving* (pp. 85–111). Hoboken, NJ: Wiley.

Losada, A., Márquez-Gonzalez, M., Knight, B. G., Yanguas, J., Sayegh, P., & Romero-Moreno, R. (2010). Psychosocial factors and caregivers' distress: Effects of familism and dysfunctional thoughts. *Aging & Mental Health, 14,* 193–202. doi:10.1080/13607860903167838

Mace, N., & Rabins, P. (2006). *The 36-hour day: A family guide to caring for persons with Alzheimer disease, related dementing illnesses, and memory loss in later life* (4th ed.). Baltimore, MD: The Johns Hopkins University Press.

Malouff, J. M., Thorsteinsson, E., & Schutte, N. (2007). The efficacy of problem-solving therapy in reducing mental and physical health problems: A meta-analysis. *Clinical Psychology Review, 27,* 46–57. doi:10.1016/j.cpr.2005.12.005

Marshall, W. M., Seal, C., & Vanatta-Perry, L. (2007). A primer for legal proceedings. In S. H. Qualls & M. A. Smyer (Eds.), *Changes in decision-making capacity in older adults: Assessment and intervention* (pp. 121–144). Hoboken, NJ: Wiley.

McDaniel, S. H. (1995). *Counseling families with chronic illness.* Alexandria, VA: American Counseling Association.

McDaniel, S. H., Campbell, T. L., Hepworth, J., & Lorenz, A. (2005). *Family-oriented primary care* (2nd ed.). New York, NY: Springer.

McDaniel, S. H., Hepworth, J., & Doherty, W. J. (1992). *Medical family therapy: A biopsychosocial approach to families with health problems.* New York, NY: Basic Books.

McDaniel, S. H., Hepworth, J., & Doherty, W. J. (1997). *The shared experience of illness.* New York, NY: Basic Books.

McGoldrick, M., Gerson, R., & Petry, S. (2008). *Genograms: Assessment and intervention.* New York, NY: Norton.

Minuchin, S. (1974). *Families and family therapy.* Cambridge, MA: Harvard University Press.

Mittelman, M. S., Ferris, S. H., Steinberg, G., Shulman, E., Mackell, J. A., Ambinder, A., & Cohen, J. (1993). An intervention that delays institutionalization of Alzheimer's Disease patients: Treatment of spouse-caregivers. *The Gerontologist, 33,* 730–740. doi:10.1093/geront/33.6.730

Mittelman, M. S., Roth, D. L., Clay, O. J., & Haley, W. E. (2007). Preserving health of Alzheimer caregivers: Impact of a spouse caregiver intervention. *The American Journal of Geriatric Psychiatry, 15,* 780–789. doi:10.1097/JGP.0b013e31805d858a

Mittelman, M. S., Roth, D. L., Coon, D. W., & Haley, W. E. (2004). Sustained benefit of supportive intervention for depressive symptoms in caregivers of patients with Alzheimer's disease. *The American Journal of Psychiatry, 161,* 850–856. doi:10.1176/appi.ajp.161.5.850

Montgomery, R. J. V., & Kosloski, K. (2011). Caregiving as a process of changing identity: Implications for caregiver support. *Generations, 33,* 47–52.

Moye, J., & Braun, M. (2007). Assessment of medical consent capacity and independent living. In S. H. Qualls & M. A. Smyer (Eds.), *Changes in decision-making capacity in older adults: Assessment and intervention* (pp. 205–236). Hoboken, NJ: Wiley.

Mukamel, D. B., Temkin-Greener, H., Delavan, R., Peterson, D. R., Gross, D., Kunitz, S., & Franklin Williams, T. (2006). Team performance and risk-adjusted health outcomes in the Program of All-Inclusive Care for the Elderly (PACE). *The Gerontologist, 46,* 227–237. doi:10.1093/geront/46.2.227

National Alliance for Caregiving. (2009). *Caregiving in the U.S.* Retrieved from http://www.caregiving.org/data/Caregiving_in_the_US_2009_full_report.pdf

National Alliance for Caregiving. (2011). *What made you think Mom had Alzheimer's?* Washington, DC: Author.

Nerenberg, L. (2008). *Elder abuse prevention: Emerging trends and promising strategies.* New York, NY: Springer.

Nezu, A. (2004). Problem solving and behavior therapy revisited. *Behavior Therapy, 35,* 1–33. doi:10.1016/S0005-7894(04)80002-9

Nezu, D., Palmatier, A., & Nezu, A. (2004). Problem-solving therapy for caregivers. In E. C. Chang, T. J. D'Zurilla, & L. J. Sanna (Eds.), *Social problem solving: Theory, research, and training* (pp. 223–238). Washington, DC: American Psychological Association. doi:10.1037/10805-013

Nichols, L. O., & Martindale-Adams, J. (2006). The decisive moment: Caregivers' recognition of dementia. *Clinical Gerontologist, 30,* 39–52. doi:10.1300/J018v30n01_04

O'Neill, P. O., & Flanagan, E. A. (1998). Elderly customers are a significant market—but may need special protection. *Journal of Retail Banking Services, 20,* 25–33.

Orfei, M. D., Robinson, R. G., Bria, P., Caltagirone, C., & Spalletta, G. (2008). Unawareness of illness in neuropsychiatric disorders: Phenomenological certainty versus etiopathogenic vagueness. *The Neuroscientist, 14,* 203–222. doi:10.1177/1073858407309995

Pearlin, L. I., Mullan, J. T., Semple, S. J., & Skaff, M. M. (1990). Caregiving and the stress process: An overview of concepts and their measures. *The Gerontologist, 30,* 583–594. doi:10.1093/geront/30.5.583

Pfeiffer, E. (1999). Stages of caregiving. *American Journal of Alzheimer's Disease, 14,* 125–127. doi:10.1177/153331759901400207

Pinquart, M., & Sörensen, S. (2005a). Caregiving distress and psychological health of caregivers. In K. V. Oxington (Ed.), *Psychology of stress* (pp. 165–206). Hauppauge, NY: Nova Biomedical Books.

Pinquart, M., & Sörensen, S. (2005b). Ethnic differences in stressors, resources, and psychological outcomes of family caregiving: A meta-analysis. *The Gerontologist, 45,* 90–106. doi:10.1093/geront/45.1.90

Pinquart, M., & Sörensen, S. (2006). Helping caregivers of persons with dementia: Which interventions work and how large are their effects? *International Psychogeriatrics, 18,* 577–595. doi:10.1017/S1041610206003462

Pinquart, M., & Sörensen, S. (2007). Correlates of physical health of informal caregivers: A meta-analysis. *The Journals of Gerontology, Series B: Psychological Sciences, 62,* P126–P137. doi:10.1093/geronb/62.2.P126

Pruchno, R. A., Blow, F. C., & Smyer, M. A. (1984). Life events and interdependent lives: Implications for research and intervention. *Human Development, 27,* 31–41. doi:10.1159/000272901

Qualls, S. H. (2007a). Clinical interventions for decision making with impaired persons. In S. H. Qualls & M. A. Smyer (Eds.), *Changes in decision-making capacity in older adults: Assessment and intervention* (pp. 271–298). Hoboken, NJ: Wiley.

Qualls, S. H. (2007b). Decision-making capacity: The players. In S. H. Qualls & M. A. Smyer (Eds.), *Changes in decision-making capacity in older adults: Assessment and intervention* (pp. 109–120). Hoboken, NJ: Wiley.

Qualls, S. H. (2008). Caregiver family therapy. In B. Knight & K. Laidlaw (Eds.), *Handbook of emotional disorders in older adults* (pp. 183–209). Oxford, England: Oxford University Press.

Qualls, S. H., & Noecker, T. L. (2009). Caregiver family therapy for conflicted families. In S. H. Qualls & S. H. Zarit (Eds.), *Aging families and caregiving: A clinician's guide to research, practice, and technology* (pp. 155–188). Hoboken, NJ: Wiley.

Rehab General Neuro-Musculo Best Practice Team. (2004). *Rehabilitation best practice standards: Functional standard number 13, IADL.* Retrieved from http://www.viha.ca/NR/rdonlyres/B9279155-0172-40E7-86F4-80D026B68855/0/iadl1_stnd_13_doc.pdf

Reinhard, S. C., Kassner, E., & Houser, A. (2011). How the Affordable Care Act can help states toward a high-performing system of long-term services and supports. *Health Affairs, 30,* 447–453. doi:10.1377/hlthaff.2011.0099

Roberto, K. A. (1999). Making critical health care decisions for older adults: Consensus among family members. *Family Relations, 48,* 167–175. doi:10.2307/585080

Robinson, B. (1983). Validation of a Caregiver Strain Index. *Journal of Gerontology, 38,* 344–348.

Rodgers, R. H., & White, J. W. (1993). Family development theory. In P. G. Boss, W. J. Doherty, R. LaRossa, W. R. Schumm, & S. K. Steinmetz (Eds.), *Sourcebook of family theories and methods* (pp. 225–257). New York, NY: Plenum. doi:10.1007/978-0-387-85764-0_10

Rolland, J. S. (1994). *Families, illness, and disability: An integrative treatment model.* New York, NY: Basic Books.

Sahler, O. J. Z., Fairclough, D. L., Phipps, S., Mulhern, R. K., Dolgin, M. J., Noll, R. B., . . . Butler, R. W. (2005). Using problem-solving skills training to reduce negative affectivity in mothers of children with newly diagnosed cancer: Report of a multisite randomized trial. *Journal of Consulting and Clinical Psychology, 73,* 272–283. doi:10.1037/0022-006X.73.2.272

Schulz, R. (1995). Psychiatric and physical morbidity effects of dementia caregiving: Prevalence, correlates, and causes. *The Gerontologist, 35,* 771–791. doi:10.1093/geront/35.6.771

Schulz, R., & Beach, S. R. (1999). Caregiving as a risk factor for mortality: The caregiver health effects study. *Journal of the American Medical Association, 282,* 2215–2219. doi:10.1001/jama.282.23.2215

Schulz, R., & Martire, L. M. (2004). Family caregiving of persons with dementia: Prevalence, health effects, and support strategies. *The American Journal of Geriatric Psychiatry, 12,* 240–249. doi:10.1176/appi.ajgp.12.3.240

Seaburn, D., Landau-Stanton, J., & Horwitz, S. (1995). Core techniques in family therapy. In R. H. Mikesell, D. D. Lusterman, & S. H. McDaniel (Eds.), *Integrating family therapy: Handbook of family psychology and systems theory* (pp. 5–26). Washington, DC: American Psychological Association Press. doi:10.1037/10172-001

Seltzer, M. M., Greenberg, J. S., & Krauss, M. W. (1995). A comparison of coping strategies of aging mothers of adults with mental illness or mental retardation. *Psychology and Aging, 10,* 64–75. doi:10.1037/0882-7974.10.1.64

Settersten, R. A., & Hagestad, G. O. (1996). What's the latest? Cultural age deadlines for family transitions. *The Gerontologist, 36,* 178–188. doi:10.1093/geront/36.2.178

Shifren, K. (2008). Early caregiving: Perceived parental relations and current social support. *Journal of Adult Development, 15*(3–4), 160–168. doi:10.1007/s10804-008-9047-6

Sörensen, S., & Conwell, Y. (2011). Issues in dementia caregiving: Effects on mental and physical health, intervention strategies, and research needs. *The American Journal of Geriatric Psychiatry, 19,* 491–496. doi:10.1097/JGP.0b013e31821c0e6e

Stephens, M. A. P., & Franks, M. (2009). All in the family: Providing care to chronically ill and disabled older adults. In S. H. Qualls & S. H. Zarit (Eds.), *Aging families and caregiving* (pp. 61–84). Hoboken, NY: Wiley.

Teri, L., Truax, P., Logsdon, R., Uomoto, J., Zarit, S., & Vitaliano, P. P. (1992). Assessment of behavioral problems in dementia: The Revised Memory and Behavior Problems Checklist. *Psychology and Aging, 7,* 622–631. doi:10.1037/0882-7974.7.4.622

Tighe, S. K., Leoutsakos, J.-M. S., Carlson, M. C., Onyike, C. U., Samus, Q., Baker, A., . . . Lyketsos, C. G. (2008). The association between activity participation and time to discharge in the assisted living setting. *International Journal of Geriatric Psychiatry, 23,* 586–591. doi:10.1002/gps.1940

Tueth, M. J. (2000). Exposing financial exploitation of impaired elderly persons. *The American Journal of Geriatric Psychiatry, 8,* 104–111.

Visser, P. J., & Verhey, F. R. J. (2008). Mild cognitive impairment as predictor for Alzheimer's disease in clinical practice: Effect of age and diagnostic criteria. *Psychological Medicine, 38,* 113–122. doi:10.1017/S0033291707000554

Vitaliano, P. P., Young, H. M., & Zhang, J. (2004). Is caregiving a risk factor for illness? *Current Directions in Psychological Science, 13,* 13–16. doi:10.1111/j.0963-7214.2004.01301004.x

Walsh, F. (Ed.). (2003). *Normal family processes: Growing diversity and complexity* (3rd ed.). New York, NY: Guilford Press. doi:10.4324/9780203428436

Watzlawick, P., Beavin, J. H., & Jackson, D. D. (1967). *Pragmatics of human communication.* New York, NY: Norton.

Watzlawick, P., Weakland, J. H., & Fisch, R. (1974). *Change: Principles of problem formation and problem resolution.* New York, NY: Norton.

Weiss, R. S. (1973). *Loneliness: The experience of emotional and social isolation.* Cambridge, MA: MIT Press.

Wilber, K. H., & Reynolds, S. L. (1997). Introducing a framework for defining financial abuse of the elderly. *Journal of Elder Abuse & Neglect, 8,* 61–80. doi:10.1300/J084v08n02_06

Williams, J. H., Drinka, T. J. K., Greenburg, J. R., Farrell-Holton, J., Euhardy, R., & Schram, M. (1991). Development and testing of the Assessment of Living Skills and Resources (ALSAR) in elderly community-dwelling veterans. *The Gerontologist, 31,* 84–91. doi:10.1093/geront/31.1.84

Williams, M., & Lewis, H. (2009). A platform for intervention and research on family communication in elder care. In S. H. Qualls &

S. H. Zarit (Eds.), *Aging families and caregiving* (pp. 269–286). Hoboken, NJ: Wiley.

Wood, S., & Tanius, B. E. (2007). Impact of dementia on decision-making abilities. In S. H. Qualls & M. A. Smyer (Eds.), *Changes in decision-making capacity in older adults: Assessment and intervention* (pp. 91–106). Hoboken, NJ: Wiley.

World Health Organization. (2011). *World health statistics.* Geneva, Switzerland: Author.

Yesavage, J. A., Brink, T. L., Rose, T. L., Lum, O., Huang, V., Adey, M., & Leirer, V.O. (1982–1983). Development and validation of a geriatric depression screening scale: A preliminary report. *Journal of Psychiatric Research, 17,* 37–49. doi:10.1016/0022-3956(82)90033-4

Zarit, S. H. (2009). Empirically supported treatment for family caregivers. In S. H. Qualls & S. H. Zarit (Eds.), *Aging families and caregiving* (pp. 131–154). Hoboken, NJ: Wiley.

Zarit, S. H., & Femia, E. E. (2008). A future for family care and dementia intervention research? Challenges and strategies. *Aging & Mental Health, 12,* 5–13. doi:10.1080/13607860701616317

Zarit, S. H., Orr, N. K., & Zarit, J. M. (1985). *Families under stress: Caring for the patient with Alzheimer's disease and related disorders.* New York, NY: New York University Press.

Zarit, S. H., Reever, K. E., & Bach-Peterson, J. (1980). Relatives of the impaired elderly: Correlations of feeling of burden. *The Gerontologist, 20,* 649–655. doi:10.1093/geront/20.6.649

Zeiss, A., Gallagher-Thompson, D., Lovett, S., Rose, J., & McKibbin, C. (1999). Self-efficacy as a mediator of caregiver coping: Development and testing of an assessment model. *Journal of Clinical Geropsychology, 5,* 221–230. doi:10.1023/A:1022955817074

Index

About the Authors

Sara Honn Qualls, PhD, is the Kraemer Family Professor of Aging Studies, professor of psychology, and director of the Gerontology Center at the University of Colorado, Colorado Springs (UCCS). She led the development of the doctoral program in clinical psychology that emphasizes geropsychology at the University of Colorado Aging Center, where trainees provide mental health and family interventions for older adults. She also founded the collaboration between UCCS and the Palisades at Broadmoor Park, a privately owned senior residential community where faculty and students provide services and conduct research.

Dr. Qualls has published several books in geropsychology, including *Aging and Mental Health,* and a clinical geropsychology series for clinicians. Her research currently focuses on the family caregiver therapy intervention, technology interventions designed to produce prosocial behavior in older adults and families, and senior housing wellness models. Within the American Psychological Association, she served on the Presidential Task Force on Caregiving, which produced a Family Caregiver Briefcase of resources for psychologists in 2010, and she chaired the Committee on Aging in 2011.

Ashley A. Williams, PhD, is the director of behavioral health at the Resource Exchange, a nonprofit agency serving individuals with intellectual and developmental disabilities. She provides behavioral therapy in the Developmental Disabilities Health Center, an innovative, integrated primary care setting. She provides services to caregivers and parents of persons with developmental disabilities and trains and supervises interns and practicum students.

Dr. Williams is also a research professor at the Gerontology Center at the University of Colorado, Colorado Springs. In this position, she completed a validation study of a computerized program to detect cognitive impairment and mental health problems in a primary care setting and conducts research on caregiver interventions. She recently completed a 3-year term as a co-convener of the Special Interest Group on Developmental Disabilities at the Gerontological Society of America's annual meetings.